The Axis Vertebra

Demetrios S. Korres

Editor

The Axis Vertebra

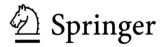 Springer

Demetrios S. Korres
Emeritus Professor in Orthopedics
Athens University Medical School
Athens
Greece

ISBN 978-88-470-5231-4   ISBN 978-88-470-5232-1   (eBook)
DOI 10.1007/978-88-470-5232-1
Springer Milan Heidelberg New York Dordrecht London

Library of Congress Control Number: 2013932552

Printed on acid-free paper

Springer is part of Springer Science+Business Media (www.springer.com)

Preface

*Χρή δέ πρ ῶτον μέν γιγνώσκειν τήν φύσιν τῆς ῥάχιος, οἵ η τίς
ἐστίν· ἐς πολλά γάρ νουσήματα προσδέοι ἄν αὐτῆς....*
Ἱπποκράτους «περί ἄρθρων» XLV

*One should first get knowledge of the structure of the
Spine; for this is also requisite for many diseases....*
Hippocrates "On Joints" XLV

The cervical spine represents a quite vulnerable area of the human skeleton, involved in many traumatic and medical conditions. Therefore, understanding the problems and managing the patients with disorders of the cervical spine is challenging. Of all the cervical vertebrae, the second has a particular interest. The second cervical vertebra is called "axis" or "epistropheus", names derived from the ancient Greek άξων (axon) or επιστροφεύς (epistrofefs) that indicate its function: it forms the pivot upon which the first cervical vertebra (the atlas), which carries the head, rotates. The most distinctive characteristic of this bone is the strong odontoid process (the dens), a tooth-like process that rises perpendicularly from the upper surface of axis' body.

The unique anatomy, structure, position under the head, and the wide pathology of the axis vertebra is involved was a stimulus to undertake the scientific task to write a book focused on the disorders of this particular vertebra, aiming to provide useful and concrete information with adequate illustrations for the readers.

The book is separated in four parts that include chapters written by colleagues, experts in their field. The first part provides the embryology, the anatomy, and the biomechanics of the axis. The second part includes a thorough description of the injuries of the axis, with particular emphasis to the fractures of the odontoid process, the body, and the posterior arch of the axis. In the third part, the surgical approaches to the axis are thoroughly described with explanatory illustrations. In the last part, the congenital anomalies, infections, and tumors of the axis are discussed. Each chapter addresses the specific subject, and includes detailed information, and a list of references for further reading. All chapters are appropriately illustrated with photographs, line drawings, and radiographs.

I am grateful and honored for the colleagues who have kindly contributed and shared material, thoughts, and knowledge for the writing of their chapters. I should especially thank my colleague Andreas F. Mavrogenis who assisted me throughout the preparation of this book. Finally, I wish to thank Springer Verlag editions of Italy for their help and recommendations throughout the writing and review process of *The Axis Vertebra*.

It is my hope that the readers will find this book useful from the perspective of obtaining the diagnosis and understanding the management of the patients with disorders of the axis vertebra.

Demetrios S. Korres

Contents

Part III

Part IV

Part I

Embryology

1

Dimitrios-Stergios Evangelopoulos

1.1 Embryonic Phase

Development of the body's shape begins during gastrulation, a process in which a trilaminar embryonic disk is created from a bilaminar disk. In this phase, during the 3rd week, the primitive streak, well-defined germ layers and the notochord are developed. At this time, epiblastic cells migrate from the deep surface of the primitive streak and form the embryonic endoderm [1–4]. Subsequently, cells continue to migrate from the primitive streak, creating the embryonic mesoderm. The cells that remain on the epiblastic side of the embryonic disk form the embryonic ectoderm. Cells migrating through the primitive node, at the cranial end of the primitive streak, give rise to the notochordal process that would later develop into the notochord. On both sides of the notochord, the mesoderm differentiates into paraxial, intermediate and lateral mesoderm. Paraxial mesoderm divides into paired bodies, the somites, located bilaterally of the neural tube [1, 2, 4].

The notochord and somites are the most important structures for the development of the future vertebral column [1]. Initially, 42–44 pairs of somites are formed. Each one differentiates into sclerotomes, giving rise to vertebrae and ribs and dermomyotomes for the muscles and the overlying skin. During the 4th week, mesenchymal cells of the sclerotome migrate and surround the notochord and neural tube. Once surrounded, each level separates into cranial and caudal areas between which the intervertebral disk gradually develops. Two sclerotomes are required for the proper development of a complete vertebra [1, 4]. Fusion of cranial and caudal parts of the adjacent sclerotomes creates the centrum that will further develop into the mesenchymal vertebral body. Similarly, mesenchymal cells surrounding the neural tube will give rise to the development of the vertebral arch [4].

During the 6th week, following cell migration and the onset of fusion of vertebral structures, vertebral bodies are subjected to an initial phase of chondrification followed by a second phase of ossification after the disintegration of the notochord. During this period, the developing vertebra enlarges and is subjected to structural changes, preserving its original shape. Chondrification starts at the beginning of the 6th week, at the level of the cervicothoracic junction and then proceeds cranially and caudally transforming somites into primary vertebrae. Four centers can be detected: two in each centrum that will fuse at the end of the embryonic period, contributing to the development of the vertebral body and two at the isthmus, bilaterally, for the development of vertebral arches. Fusion between body and arches occurs at the end of the 8th week at the initiation of the ossification phase [1–5].

D.-S. Evangelopoulos (✉)
Third Department of Orthopedic Surgery,
University of Athens, 48, Lamesou Street,
15669 Papagos, Athens, Attika, Greece
e-mail: ds.evangelopoulos@gmail.com

D. S. Korres (ed.), *The Axis Vertebra*,
DOI: 10.1007/978-88-470-5232-1_1, © Springer-Verlag Italia 2013

1.2   Prenatal Period

During this period, ossification centers can be found in three main vertebral regions: one in the centrum and one on each side of the vertebral arch [4, 5]. The vertebral body will articulate with the vertebral arch at the neurocentral joints at birth. Fusion occurs later on, between the age of 5 and 8 years. The two pieces of the arch begin to fuse during the first year of life with complete fusion occurring by the age of 6 years [1, 4]. The five secondary ossification centers that will form after birth, as described by Moore et al. are one for the tip of each transverse process, one for the extremity of the spinous process, one for the upper and one for the lower surface of the body (Fig. 1.1) [1, 2, 4]. Ossified bone deriving from the secondary centers will contribute to the formation of growth plates. Absence and/or asymmetry of growth plates is believed to contribute to the development of congenital defects. Additionally, defects in both chondrification and ossification may lead to the development of known congenital abnormalities.

Molecular signals from the notochord are responsible for the differentiation, chondrification and ossification of the vertebrae [6]. The notochord along with several genes as well as the involved signaling pathways enables the proper development of the vertebrae and the nervous system.

Torklus et al. accurately described the development of the axis body. The authors reported a detailed description on the five centers of ossification of the axis vertebra. The

process initiates at the second fetal month, through perichondral ossification, on the two posterolateral centers from the arch of the axis [6, 7]. Their anterior expansion contributes to the ossification of the vertebral body. At the fifth fetal month, one median ossification center gives rise to a significant section of the vertebral body while two primary ossification centers arising cranially to the median center give rise to the dens axis through cranially directed ossification, remaining separated from the body's ossification center through subdental synchondrosis.

The odontoid process represents a distinct process lying separated cranially to the body of the axis since its primitive development. Wang et al. reported that this synchondrosis is restricted to the medial border of the superior articular facets of the axis [8]. However, in the study of Torklus et al. during development, the odontoid process together with the subdental synchondrosis is shown to countersink into the corpus of the axis as being an independent anatomical structure, the basis of the odontoid process [5, 7]. Several authors concluded that the syndesmosis represents a bipolar growth zone located below the level of the atlantoaxial articulation, contributing to the height of the base of the dens and the vertebral body [9–11]. Highlighting these results, Cokluk et al., in their MRI study on the upper cervical spine of pediatric and adult patients, demonstrated the independent structure of the odontoid process and recognized the remnants of the subdental syndesmosis as a hypointense ring located well below the level of the superior articulating facets [12].

The distinct development of the odontoid process compared to the body of the axis necessitates reconsideration of the Anderson-D'Alonso classification of odontoid process fractures [13, 14]. Additionally, the base of the odontoid process and the subdental region, apart from the unique anatomy, distinct anatomical features of the region and different origin, demonstrates delayed ossification, compared to the body and the neck of the odontoid process, leading to altered age-related structural and biomechanical properties (Fig. 1.2) [14]. For the above-mentioned, to achieve optimal treatment

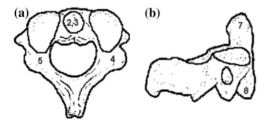

Fig. 1.1 Development of the axis. The five primary [Fig. 1.1a: body (*1*), dens (*2, 3*), lateral masses (*4, 5*)] and two secondary [Fig. 1.1b: inferior epiphyseal plate (*6*), Bergmann's (*7*)] centers

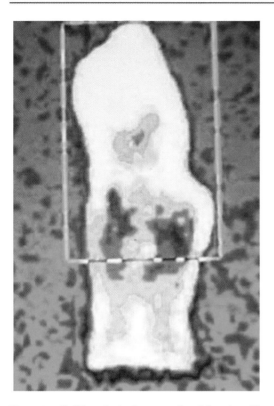

Fig. 1.2 pQ-CT analysis demonstrating delayed ossification of the basis of the dens and the subdental region, compared to the body and the neck of the dens

and allow accurate prognosis, fractures at the base of the odontoid process should be considered as a separate trauma entity in the different fracture classification systems and not as an extension of fracture lines from the body of the axis.

References

1. Korres DS (1999) Cervical spine: traumatology-pathology. Litsas Medical Publications, Athens

2. Sherk HH, Parke WW (1989) Developmental anatomy. Cervical spine, 2nd edn. J. Lippincott, Philadelphia

3. Wackenheim A (1989) Imaginerie du rachis cervical. Springer, Berlin

4. Kaplan KM, Spivak JM, Bendo JA (2005) Embryology of the spine and associated congenital abnormalities. Spine J 5:564–576

5. Torklus D, Gehle W (1968) Das Os odontoideum als Okzipitalwirbelmanifestation. Radil Clin Biol 37:321

6. Bailey DK (1952) The normal cervical spine in infants and children. Radiology 59:712–719

7. Torklus D, Gehle W (1969) Neue Perspektiven der Entwicklungsstorungen der oberen Halswirbelsaule. Z Orthop 105:78

8. Wang XP, Deng ZC, Liang ZJ, Tu YU (2008) Response to reply to the letter to the editor concerning Gebauer et al.: subdental synchondrosis and anatomy of the axis in aging: a histomorphometric study on 30 autopsy cases. Eur Spine J 17:1771–1774

9. Gebauer M, Barvencik F, Beil FT, Lohse C, Pogoda P, Puschel K, Rueger JM, Amling M (2007) Subdental synchondrosis: computed tomographic and histologic investigation on morphological aspects of fracture of the base of the dens in 36 human axis specimens. Unfallchirurg 110:97–103

10. Gebauer M, Amling M (2008) The development of the axis vertebra: the key to a topographic classification of dens fractures. Eur Spine J 17:1775–1777

11. Amling M, Hahn M, Wening VJ, Grote HJ, Delling J (1994) The microarchitecture of the axis as the predisposing factor for fracture of the base of the odontoid process. A histomorphometric analysis of twenty-two autopsy specimens. J Bone Joint Surg Am 76:1840–1846

12. Coklul C, Aydin K, Rakunt C, Iyigum O, Onder A (2006) The borders of the odontoid process of C2 in adults and in children including the estimation of odontoid/body ratio. Eur Spine J 15:292–298

13. Anderson LD, D'Alonzo RT (1974) Fractures of the odontoid process of the axis. J Bone Joint Surg Am 56:1663–1674

14. Korres DS, Karachalios T, Roidis N, Lycomitros V, Spiliopoulou CA, Lyritis G (2004) Structural properties of the axis studied in cadaveric specimens. Clin Orthop 418:134–140

Anatomy

2

Andrés Combalia

A thorough knowledge of the anatomy of the cervical spine is essential for the performance of surgical procedures. Recent qualitative and quantitative studies using cadaver dissection, computed tomography, and magnetic resonance imaging have continued to add to our knowledge of the dimension of and the clinically relevant relations between cervical spine structures. This chapter discusses the normal anatomy of the second cervical vertebra and its relations.

2.1 Osseous Components of Craniocervical Junction

The first (atlas) and second (axis) cervical vertebrae are considered atypical compared with those of the lower cervical spine. Atlas lacks a body and a spinous process. It is a ring-like structure consisting of two lateral masses connected by a short anterior arch and a longer posterior arch. It is the widest cervical vertebra, with its anterior arch approximately half as long as its posterior arch (Fig. 2.1). Located in the midline of the anterior arch is the anterior tubercle for the attachment of the anterior

A. Combalia (✉)
Orthopaedic Surgery and Traumatology, Hospital Clínic, University of Barcelona and Department Human Anatomy, Faculty of Medicine, University of Barcelona, Villarroel 170, Barcelona, 08036, Spain
e-mail: combalia@clinic.ub.es

longitudinal ligament and the longus colli muscles. The posterior arch corresponds to the lamina of the other vertebrae. On its upper surface is a wide groove for the vertebral artery and the first cervical nerve. In 1–15 % of the population, a bony arch may form, thereby converting this groove into the arcuate foramen, through which passes the same structures [1–3]. On the posterior arch is a posterior tubercle for attachment of the ligamentum nuchae. The lower surface is notched, which contributes to the formation of the C2 intervertebral foramen. The lateral masses of the atlas give rise to a superior and inferior articular facet. The transverse process is larger than that of other cervical vertebrae and is composed solely of a posterior tubercle that, with the costotransverse bar that attaches to the lateral mass, contains the foramen transversarium. An important anatomic feature of the atlas is the inward projection of a prominent tubercle of bone on each side cranial and medially to the lateral masses. These structures give rise to the transverse ligament that keeps the dens confined to the anterior third of the atlantal ring. This relation allows free rotation of the atlas on the dens and axis and provides, together with the other ligaments for a stable configuration in flexion, extension and lateral bending [4].

The axis is also known as the epitropheus. It is characterized by a dens or odontoid process that projects upward from the vertebral body to articulate with the posterior aspect of the anterior arch of the atlas (Fig. 2.2). The dimensions

D. S. Korres (ed.), *The Axis Vertebra*,
DOI: 10.1007/978-88-470-5232-1_2, © Springer-Verlag Italia 2013

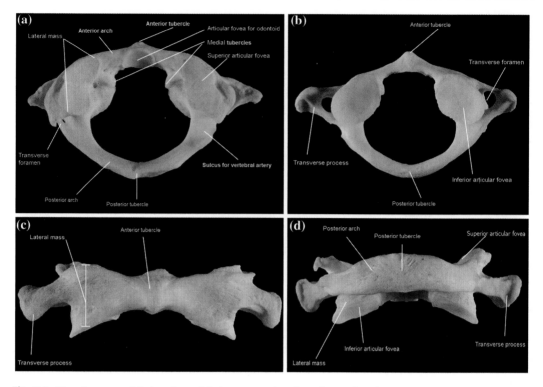

Fig. 2.1 The atlas: **a** cranial view, **b** caudal view, **c** anterior view, **d** posterior view

of the dens are highly variable: Its mean height is 37.8 mm, its external transverse diameter is 9.3 mm, internal transverse diameter is 4.5 mm, mean anteroposterior external diameter is 10.5 mm, and internal diameter is 6.2 mm [5]. Lateral to the dens, the body has a facet for the lower surface of atlas' lateral mass, which is large, slightly convex, and faces upward and outward. It is not a true superior articular process because the articular surface arises directly from the body and pedicle lateral to the dens. The zone between the lamina and the lateral mass is not well defined and comprises a large pedicle/isthmus that is 10 mm long and 8 mm wide [6]. It projects superiorly and medially in an anterior direction. The lower surface of the lateral mass has a forward-facing facet that articulates with the superior articular process of C3. Axis' pedicle/isthmus plays an important role regarding screw purchase for spinal fixation. The location of axis' pedicle remains a subject of controversy. Although some authors have reported that the pedicle connects the vertebral body to the superior articular process [7, 8], others have defined the pedicle as the portion beneath and posterior to the superior facet [9–12]. There is a confusion regarding the terminology of these structures. A pedicle is a portion of the vertebrae connecting the ventral and dorsal elements. Although this is valid for all subaxial vertebrae, the axis' pedicles are anatomically unique. Although the superior articular process is a posterior element of the vertebra (i.e., posterior to vertebral body in the axial plane) in all subaxial vertebrae, an inspection of the axis reveals that its superior articular process is not anatomically posterior to the vertebral body. Naderi et al. [13] studied 160 axis' pedicles (80 dry vertebrae). The isthmus (pars interarticularis) and the pedicle are distinct structures. The axis does not have an isolated pedicle, which can be observed in the subaxial vertebrae. There exists a complex containing the pedicle inferiorly and the isthmus superiorly. Whereas the isthmus connects the superior and inferior articular processes, the true pedicle

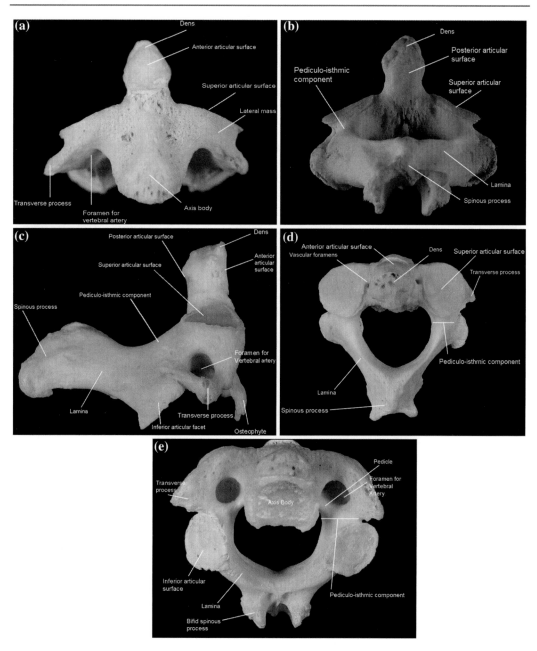

Fig. 2.2 The axis: **a** anterior view, **b** posterior view, **c** lateral view, **d** cranial view, and **e** caudal view

connects the lateral mass and inferior articular process to the vertebral body.

The pedicle of the axis is covered by the facet joint and integrated with the isthmus. Therefore, for Naderi et al. [13], it is more appropriate to term these two components as the pediculoisthmic components (PIC) due to the fact that although both are distinct structures they are closely integrated. The axial PIC is posterolateral to the vertebral body, medial to the transverse foramen, originates posterolaterally from the lateral mass and inferior articular process junction, and ends anteromedially at the vertebral body–odontoid process junction. It is grooved laterally by the transverse foramen. The axis' isthmus covers the pedicle. The heights of the right and the left PICs in the Naderi et al. study were 10.3 ± 1.6 and 9.9 ± 1.5 mm, respectively. The posterior part of the superior aspect of the PIC is wider than the anterior portion. The widths of the posterosuperior aspect of the PIC were 11.1 ± 2 and 11 ± 1.7 mm on the right and left sides, whereas the widths of the antero-superior aspect of the PIC were 7.9 ± 1.7 and 8.5 ± 1.6 mm, respectively. The inferior widths of this component were 6.0 ± 1.5 and 5.5 ± 1.3 mm on the right and left sides, respectively. The lengths of the component were 28.8 ± 2.9 mm on the right and 28.8 ± 3.4 mm on the left side [13]. The PIC exhibits a lateral-to-medial angle and an inferior-to-superior angle. Its axial angles were 28.4° ± 2.5° and 28.6° ± 2.2° on the right and left sides, respectively; its sagittal angles were 18.8° ± 2.1° and 18.8° ± 1.7°, respectively. In summary, axis' pedicle can be seen in the inferior aspect of the vertebra, and it connects posterior vertebral elements (i.e., the lateral mass and inferior articular process) to the axial body. The isthmus or pars interarticularis drapes the pedicle.

The laminae of the axis are thick, and the spinous process is large and bifid. The transverse process ends in a single tubercle and contains a foramen transversarium. Cassinelli et al. [14] measured the laminar thickness (LT) in the narrowest laminar section in American populations and reported that more than 70.6 % of the specimens they studied had a LT > 5 mm. Mean laminar thickness was 5.77 ± 1.31 mm; 92.6 % had a thickness ≥4.0 mm. The spinolaminar angle was 48.59° ± 5.42°. Ma et al. [15] evaluated axis' lamina in Asian population. A total of 83.3 % specimens had bilateral laminar thicknesses ≥4.0 mm and a spinous process height ≥9.0 mm. Wright in 2004 [16] described a new technique for fixation involving bilateral, crossing laminar screws. More than 99 % of specimens in the Cassinelli study had an estimated screw length of at least 20 mm. Gender had a significant effect on all of the measurements studied. It is not likely, however, that all of these differences are clinically significant.

White males had the thickest laminae, while white females had the thinnest. Laminar thickness was 0.46 mm (8.3 %) less in females than in males. There was no statistical effect of patient race, height, or weight on any of the measurements [14]. Several other studies examining the LT came to similar conclusions: Most of the specimens they examined had an LT larger than the diameter of the commonly used cervical screw (3.5 mm). Although the minimum laminar thickness required to allow for safe placement of a screw was not described, there is a common idea that a thickness >5 mm with a precise screw trajectory may be acceptable [17, 18].

The spinal nerve exits posterior to the superior articular surface of the axis rather than anterior to the articular complex, as spinal nerves do at other levels. Large pediculoisthmic structures and a deeper spinal canal are two factors that allow increased mobility at the axis without cord encroachment. The density of the trabecular bone of the axis varies: It is very dense near the center of the tip of the dens and lateral masses beneath the superior articular surface, and hypodense in the area of the trabecular bone immediately beneath the dens. An area of cortical thickening on the anterior surface of the axis, known as the promontory of the axis, underlies the insertion of the anterior longitudinal ligament [19, 20].

The occipital condyles have also been thoroughly described. The occipital condyles are the paired lateral prominences of the occipital bone that form the foramen magnum together with the basioccipital segment anteriorly and the supraoccipital or squamosal segment posteriorly. The occipital condyles are commonly oval or bean shaped and slope inferiorly from lateral to medial in the coronal plane. The condyles make an angle of 25°–28° with the midsagittal plane. The occipitoatlantal articulations are cup-shaped paired joints between the convex occipital condyles and the concave superior atlantal facets. The condylar part of the occipital bone is perforated by the hypoglossal or anterior condyloid canal/foramen. Two structures travel through this canal; the hypoglossal nerve (cranial nerve

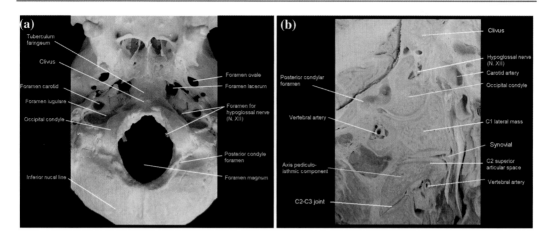

Fig. 2.3 Occipital condyles: **a** caudal view of the cranium, **b** paramedian section passing through the right occipito–atlas–axis joints

XII) exits the skull, while a meningeal branch of the ascending pharyngeal artery enters it (Fig. 2.3). Behind the occipital condyles, there is an indentation known as the condyloid fossa, which is frequently perforated by the posterior condylar foramen. And emissary vein runs through the posterior condylar canal from the sigmoid sinus. Sometimes there is also an artery which anastomoses with the posterior meningeal artery. Cranial nerves IX to XI, the inferior petrosal sinus, the internal jugular vein, and the posterior meningeal artery travel lateral to the occipital condyles in the jugular foramen.

The spinal canal is formed by sequential vertebral foramina and is triangular with rounded edges. It has a greater lateral than AP width and is more spacious in the upper cervical spine, with sagittal diameters averaging 23 mm at the atlas and 20 mm at the axis. In comparison, the average diameter from C3 through C6 ranges between 17 and 18 mm and decreases to 15 mm at C7 [21]. Thus, the cross-sectional area of the cervical spinal canal is greatest at the axis and smallest at C7.

2.2 Articulations, Biomechanics, and Ligaments

The craniovertebral junction is composed of 2 major joints: the atlantooccipital and the atlantoaxial joints. These joints are responsible for the majority of the movement of the cervical spine and operate on different biomechanical principles. The mechanical properties of the atlantooccipital joint are primarily determined by bony structures, whereas the mechanical properties of the atlantoaxial joint are mainly determined by ligamentous structures [22]. The prominent movements at the atlantooccipital joint are flexion and extension.

The various movements at this joint occur because the condyles glide in the sockets of the atlas [23]. Panjabi et al. [24] found the atlanto-occipital joint to be responsible for 27.1° of flexion and 24.9° of extension. They also noted that about 8° of axial rotation can take place at this joint, as well as minimal lateral and anteroposterior translation. Steinmetz et al. [22] reported similar values, with a mean movement of 23°–24.5° of flexion/extension, whereas axial rotation was limited to 2.4°–7.2°. They reported that flexion was limited by impingement of the odontoid process on the foramen magnum, and extension was restricted by the tectorial membrane. Lateral flexion is strongly inhibited at the atlantooccipital joint by the contralateral alar ligament [25]. The primary movement at the atlantoaxial joint is axial rotation. Steinmetz et al. [22] reported that the mean axial rotational movement was between 23.3° and 38.9°. Menezes and Traynelis [23] noted that axial rotation beyond 30°–35° can cause vertebral artery occlusion. Flexion and extension at the atlantoaxial joint range from 10.1° to 22.4° and are limited by the transverse ligament and tectorial membrane, respectively. Lateral bending is restricted to 6.7° by the contralateral alar ligament. Although these two joints function differently, they must act in unison to ensure optimal stability and mobility at the craniovertebral junction.

The atlantooccipital complex is composed of two membranous attachments between the atlas and the occiput and the two synovial atlantooccipital joints laterally. The atlantooccipital joints are formed between the superior articular facet of the atlas and the occipital condyle. These joints contain a synovial membrane and are surrounded by a capsular ligament. Also contributing to the complex are the anterior and posterior atlantooccipital membranes, connecting the anterior and posterior arch of the atlas with the corresponding margin of the foramen magnum. The anterior atlantooccipital membrane blends on its lateral edges with the capsular ligaments of the synovial joints and inferiorly with the anterior longitudinal ligament. The posterior atlantooccipital membrane blends laterally with the capsular

ligaments of the synovial joints and is pierced on each side just above the posterior arch of the atlas by the vertebral artery and the first cervical nerve (Fig. 2.4) [1].

The atlantoaxial complex is composed of three synovial joints, one median and two lateral. The lateral atlantoaxial joints consist of an encapsulated synovial joint between the inferior articular facet of the atlas and the superior articular surface of C2 (Fig. 2.3b). The capsule is reinforced posteriorly by an accessory ligament that extends from the posterior aspect of the axis superiorly and laterally to the lateral mass of the atlas [25]. This accessory atlantoaxial ligament runs at the lateral edge of the tectorial membrane and is sometimes called the "accessory part of the tectorial membrane". In a thorough description by Tsakotos et al. [26], the attachment of the tectorial membrane and the accessory atlantoaxial ligament was 0.6–1.1 cm (mean 0.9 cm) inferior to the internal opening of the anterior condylar canal (hypoglossal canal) and posterior to the cephalic attachment of the alar ligament. The maximal tension of the accessory atlantoaxial ligament was observed during rotation of the head at 5°–8°. The ligament remains lax with cervical extension and

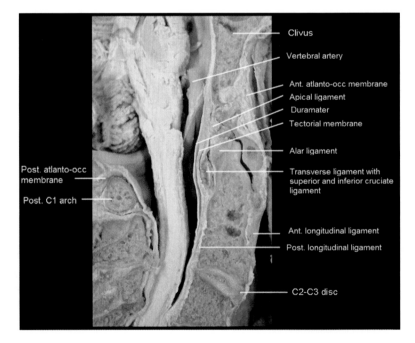

Fig. 2.4 Median section at craniovertebral junction showing atlantooccipital and atlantoaxial ligaments and anatomic structures

Clivus

Vertebral artery

Ant. atlanto-occ membrane

Apical ligament

Duramater

Tectorial membrane

Alar ligament

Transverse ligament with superior and inferior cruciate ligament

Post. atlanto-occ membrane

Post. C1 arch

Ant. longitudinal ligament

Post. longitudinal ligament

C2-C3 disc

shows no tension during cervical flexion. Its function seems to assist the alar ligament in inhibiting excessive rotation of the head, since its maximal tautness ranges from about 5° to 10°. The median atlantoaxial joint forms between the anterior arch and transverse ligament of the atlas and the dens. It is a pivot joint with synovial membrane and capsular ligaments anteriorly and posteriorly to the dens. The cruciate or cruciform ligament is composed of the transverse ligament of the atlas and the superior and inferior ligamentous extensions that connect it to the anterior edges of the foramen magnum and posterior aspect of axis' body, respectively. The transverse ligament attaches laterally to a small tubercle located on the medial aspect of the lateral mass of C1, where it blends with the lateral mass (Figs. 2.4, 2.5, 2.6). The length of the transverse ligament averages 21.9 mm. It is the largest, strongest, and thickest craniocervical ligament (mean height/thickness 6–7 mm) [25]. The transverse ligament maintains stability at the atlantoaxial joint by locking the odontoid process anteriorly against the posterior aspect of the anterior arch of the axis, and it divides the ring of the atlas into two compartments: the anterior compartment houses the odontoid process, and the posterior compartment contains primarily the spinal cord and spinal accessory nerves. The ligament also has a smooth fibrocartilaginous surface to allow the odontoid process to glide against it [23]. The tectorial membrane, epidural fat, and dura mater are located dorsal to the transverse ligament. The biomechanical data reported by Fielding et al. [27] demonstrated that the transverse ligament is the primary defense against anterior subluxation of the atlas on the axis and that it is relatively inelastic, only allowing C1 to subluxate approximately 3–5 mm before rupturing.

The axis has three other connections to the occipital bone, the apical ligament, and the alar ligaments. The apical ligament , also known as suspensory ligament, extends from the tip of the dens to the anterior edge of the foramen magnum. Panjabi et al. [24] reported the length of the apical ligament to be 23.5 mm and a 20° anterior tilt, describing the ligament as broad and fan shaped at its insertion onto the basion. They also reported the ligament as tightly adherent to the overlying tectorial membrane. The ligament runs in the triangular area between the left and right alar ligaments known as the supraodontoid space (apical cave) [28] and

Fig. 2.5 Transversal section at atlanto–odontoid joint

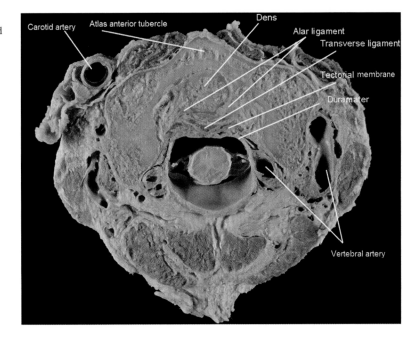

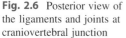

Fig. 2.6 Posterior view of the ligaments and joints at craniovertebral junction

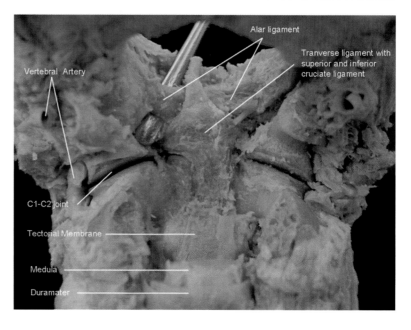

travels just posterior to the alar ligaments and just anterior to the superior portion of the cruciform ligament. In 2000, Tubbs et al. [29] conducted a cadaveric study focusing on the apical ligament and found the mean length and width to be 7.5 and 5.1 mm, respectively. They also observed the ligament to be straight at the midline with no fanning between the attachment points. They did not observe any connection between the alar and cruciform ligaments, and the tectorial membrane.

An area between the apical ligament and the superior extension of the cruciform ligament was routinely found to be filled with connective tissue, fat, and a small venous plexus. Interestingly, they found the ligament to be present in only 80 % of the cadavers. The alar ligaments extend from the tip of the dens to the medial aspects of each occipital condyle, with a small insertion also on the lateral mass of the atlas [30]. They average 10.3 mm long and run from the posterolateral aspect of the odontoid process, laterally forming an angle ranging from 125° to 210° with a mean of 154° [25]. An MR imaging study conducted by Baumert et al. [31] found that the alar ligament was oriented caudocranially in 67 % of the cases and horizontally in 33 %. The alar ligaments function as stabilizing structures of the atlantoaxial joint and act to limit axial rotation and lateral bending to the contralateral side. They are the only ligaments, except the transverse ligament, which are strong enough to stabilize the craniocervical junction and prevent anterior displacement of the atlas. If the transverse ligament ruptures, the alar ligaments become responsible for preventing atlantal subluxation. Fielding et al. [27] reported that the alar ligaments alone are not as strong as the transverse ligament. The alar ligaments serve as secondary restrictions of the atlas to anterior shift [27]. Following the rupture of the transverse ligament, a mean force of 72 kg was needed to stretch the alar ligament to create a predental space of 12 mm, and any subluxation greater than 12 mm caused the alar ligament to rupture. Similarly, Dvorak et al. [30] noted that the transverse ligament could withstand a load of 350 N, whereas the alar ligament could only withstand 200 N before rupturing. The alar ligament limits the axial rotation on the contralateral side to about 90°. Sometimes there is a ligamentous connection between the base of the dens and the anterior arch of the atlas (anterior atlantodental ligament) . In a recent work by Tubbs et al. [32], the anterior atlantodental ligament was found in 81.3 % of 16 specimens dissected. The attachment of each ligament was consistent and travelled between the base of the anterior dens to the posterior aspect of the anterior arch of the atlas in the midline and just inferior to the fovea dentis. The ligament was roughly $4 \times 4 \times 4$ mm in all specimens.

The tectorial membranes extend from the posterior body of the axis and the posterior longitudinal ligament to the upper surface of the basilar portion of the occipital bone and the anterior aspect of the foramen magnum. This membrane covers all other occipitoaxial ligaments as well as the dens. Thus, anterior to the spinal canal at the level of the craniocervical junction, the ligaments are arranged with the anterior atlantooccipital membrane most anteriorly followed (in an anterior-to-posterior direction) by the apical, the alar, and the cruciate and, most posteriorly, the tectorial [1]. The tectorial membrane firmly adhered to the cranial base and body of the axis but not to the posterior odontoid process [24]. Other ligaments have been remembered and described in recent publications by Tubbs et al. [25, 33].

The transverse occipital ligament (TOL) is a small accessory ligament of the craniovertebral junction that is located posterosuperior to the alar ligaments and odontoid process. It attaches to the inner aspect of the occipital condyles, posterosuperior to the alar ligament, superior to the transverse ligament, and extends horizontally across the foramen magnum. Tubbs et al. [33] have identified it in 7 (77.8 %) of 9 human cadavers. Dvorak et al. [34] stated that the TOL was only present in about 10 % of the population, whereas Lang [35] identified the TOL in approximately 40 % of their specimens. The discrepancies in the occurrence of the TOL in specimens could be due to the proximity and similar morphology to the alar ligament. Clinically, the TOL may be encountered during a transoral odontoidectomy.

The Barkow's ligament, rarely described, is a horizontal band attaching onto the anteromedial aspect of the occipital condyles anterior to the attachment of the alar ligaments. This ligament is located just anterior to the superior aspect of the dens with fibers traveling anterior to the alar

ligaments, but there is no attachment to these structures. Tubbs et al. [36] found the ligament to be present in 12 (92.3 %) of 13 cadavers, observing an attachment between the Barkow's ligament and the anterior atlantooccipital membrane at the midline in 9 specimens (75 %).

The articulation between the axis and the third vertebra has the same anatomic characteristics of the subaxial cervical spine. The bodies of the cervical vertebrae are connected by two longitudinal ligaments and the intervertebral disks. The anterior longitudinal ligament is a broad, thick ligament that runs longitudinally anterior to the vertebral body and disk. It is joined loosely to the periosteum of the anterior vertebral bodies and closely to the annulus fibrosus of the anterior vertebral disk and attaches superiorly to the anterior tubercle of the atlas.

The posterior longitudinal ligament (PLL) lies within the vertebral canal on the posterior aspect of the vertebral bodies and intervertebral disks. Superiorly, it is continuous with the tectorial membrane and thus attaches to the occipital bone and anterior aspect of the foramen magnum. As it descends, it narrows behind each vertebral body but spreads out at the disk level, where it is adherent to the annulus fibrosis.

2.3   Neural Elements

The spinal cord extends from the foramen magnum above, where it is continuous with the medulla oblongata. With its surrounding meninges, it lies within the vertebral or spinal canal, which is formed by sequential vertebral foramina. The anterior wall of the spinal canal is formed by the posterior border of the intervertebral disks and cervical vertebral bodies. The lateral wall consists of the pedicles and successive intervertebral foramina, through which the spinal nerves exit. Posteriorly, the articular processes laterally and the ligamentum flavum and the lamina medially and posteriorly form the final borders of the spinal canal [1].

The first cervical spinal nerve exits between the occiput and the atlas through an orifice in the posterior atlantooccipital membrane just above the posterior arch of the atlas and posteromedial to the lateral mass of the atlas. Just beyond the dorsal root ganglion and usually just outside the intervertebral foramina, the cervical spinal nerves divide into dorsal and ventral primary rami. Its ventral primary ramus unites with the second cervical ventral primary ramus and contributes fibers to the hypoglossal nerve(this is also known as the superior root of the ansa cervicalis); the dorsal primary ramus of the C1 nerve root—also known as the suboccipital nerve—enters the suboccipital triangle and innervates the muscles of this region. It has usually no cutaneous branch [1, 37, 38].

The second cervical nerve emerges between the posterior arch of the atlas and the lamina of the axis just posterior to its lateral mass (Fig. 2.7). Its dorsal rami are much larger than its ventral rami and are the largest of all the cervical dorsal rami. The medial branch of the dorsal rami, or greater occipital nerve, runs transversely in the soft tissue dorsal to axis' lamina, turning cranial around the muscle belly of the obliquus capitis inferior muscle, piercing the semispinalis capitis muscle, and then eventually entering the scalp with the occipital artery through an opening above the aponeurotic sling between the trapezius and the stemocleidomastoid.

2.4   Vertebral Artery

The major source of blood for the osseous and neural elements of the cervical spine is the vertebral arteries, which arise from the first part of the subclavian artery medial to the scalenus anterior and ascend behind the common carotid artery between the longus colli and the scalenus anterior. They are crossed by the inferior thyroid artery and on the left by the thoracic duct. In the lower cervical region, they lie anterior to the ventral rami of the seventh and eight cervical nerves and to the transverse process of the seventh cervical vertebra. The vertebral artery usually enters the transverse foramen of C6 and ascends through the transverse foramina from C6 through the axis, in front of the ventral rami of the cervical nerves. In this region, they lie within a fibro-osseous tunnel, fixing it to adjacent structures via a trabeculated collagen network. Vertebral arteries are surrounded by a venous plexus and sympathetic nerve fibers [1, 39].

At the level of the atlas, the vertebral arteries pass through the vertebral foramen of the atlas and travel posteriorly and medially behind the lateral mass and then superiorly from the posterior arch of the atlas. As mentioned, in 1–15 % of the population, a bony arch may form, thereby

Fig. 2.7 Dissection of the posterior aspect of C1–C2 showing vertebral artery and the second cervical nerve and ganglia

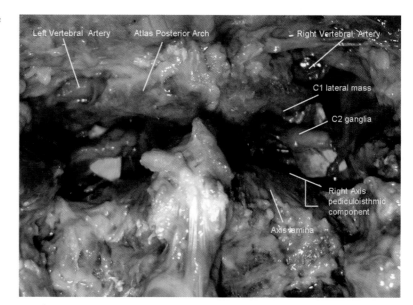

converting this groove into the arcuate foramen [3]. The arteries then pierce the posterior atlantooccipital membrane, turning anteriorly and cephalad through the foramen magnum joining to form the basilar artery. Just before forming the basilar artery, the vertebral arteries give off branches anteriorly that join to form the single anterior spinal artery. This artery runs within the anterior median fissure of the spinal cord, providing blood supply to roughly the anterior two-thirds of the spinal cord.

The posterior third of the spinal cord is supplied by two posterior spinal arteries, which arise from either the vertebral artery or the posterior inferior cerebral arteries. The nerve roots are supplied by radicular branches from the spinal arteries. Anomalies of the vertebral artery in the region of C1–C2 include fenestration or intraspinal coursing and have been found to have a prevalence of 0.3–2 % [40]. In patients having osseous anomalies at the craniovertebral junction, the frequency of vertebral artery anomalies at the extraosseous and intraosseous regions is increased. With preoperative three-dimensional computed tomography angiography, we can precisely identify the anomalous vertebral artery and reduce the risk of intraoperative injury to the vertebral artery [41].

The blood supply of the cervical vertebral bodies originates from segmental vessels off the vertebral arteries. At each level, these branches exit, passing anteriorly beneath the longus colli, supplying the anterior vertebral body and the anterior longitudinal ligament. Another branch enters the intervertebral foramina and passes anteriorly and superiorly, supplying the posterior vertebral body and the posterior longitudinal ligament. Other branches pass laterally from within the spinal canal, supplying the laminae and radicular branches to the spinal cord. The outer surface of the laminae is supplied by other branches of the vertebral artery that pass dorsally before entering the intervertebral foramina [1].

The vascular supply to the odontoid process is unique and worth mentioning. It is supplied by paired ascending anterior and posterior arteries, all of which arise from the vertebral arteries. These arteries rise along the borders of the dens

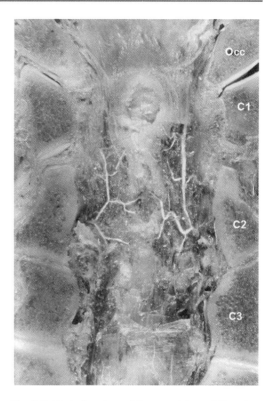

Fig. 2.8 Posterior view of the vasculature of the odontoid process (Courtesy of Prof. R. Ramón-Soler)

to form an apical arcade, which anastomoses with the carotid system via anterior and posterior horizontal arteries [39, 42, 43] (Fig. 2.8). The alar and accessory ligaments also make vascular contributions, as does an intraosseous supply from the body of the axis. Whereas the clinically observed problem of non-union of fractures of the odontoid process has been attributed to a scant blood supply, this does not appear to be the primary causative factor [4]. Venous drainage of the cervical spine occurs through internal and external venous plexi. The external veins run paired with the arteries described earlier. The internal plexus lies within the spinal canal and consists of a valveless series of epidural sinuses. This complex of veins is continuous from the cerebral sinuses distally to the pelvis. These veins are most prevalent at the vertebral bodies and thinnest at the disk spaces. They drain through the intervertebral foramina into the cava and azygos systems [39].

References

1. Heller JG, Pedlow FX, Gill SS (2005) Anatomy of the cervical spine. In: Clark CHR (ed) The cervical spine. Lippincott Williams & Wilkins, Philadelphia, pp 3–36
2. Stubbs D (1992) The arcuate foramen: variability in distribution related to race and sex. Spine 17:1502–1504
3. Young JP, Young PH, Ackermann MJ, Anderson PA, Riew KD (2005) The ponticulus posticus: implications for screw insertion into the first cervical lateral mass. J Bone Joint Surg Am Nov 87(11):2495–2498
4. Yoo JU, Hart RA (2003) Anatomy of the cervical spine. In: Emery SE, Boden SC (eds) Surgery of the cervical spine. Elsevier, Amsterdam, pp 1–10
5. Heller JG, Alson MD, Schaffler MB et al (1992) Quantitative internal dens morphology. Spine 17:861–966
6. An HS, Gordin R, Renner K (1991) Anatomic considerations for plate–screw fixation of the cervical spine. Spine 16(suppl):S548–S551
7. Benzel EC (1996) Anatomic consideration of C2 pedicle screw placement. Spine 21:2301–2302
8. Borne GM, Bedou GL, Pinaudeau M (1984) Treatment of pedicular fractures of the axis. A clinical study and screw fixation technique. J Neurosurg 60:88–93
9. Ebraheim NA, Fow J, Xu R et al (2001) The location of the pedicle and pars interarticularis in the axis. Spine 26:E34–E37
10. Ebraheim N, Rollins JR, Xu R et al (1996) Anatomic consideration of C2 pedicle screw placement. Spine 21:691–694
11. Panjabi M, Duranceau J, Goel V et al (1991) Cervical human vertebrae. Quantitative three-dimensional anatomy of the middle and lower regions. Spine 16:861–874
12. Roy-Camille R, Saillant G, Mazel C (1989) Internal fixation of the unstable cervical spine by a posterior osteosynthesis with plates and screws. In: Cervical Spine Research Society (ed) The cervical spine, 2nd edn. JB Lippincott, Philadelphia, pp 390–430
13. Naderi S, Arman C, Güvençer M, Korman E, Senoglu M, Tetik S, Arsa N (2004) An anatomical study of C2 pedicle. J Neurosurg Spine 3:306–310
14. Cassinelli EH, Lee M, Skalak A, Ahn NU, Wright NM (2006) Anatomic considerations for the placement of C2 laminar screws. Spine 24:2767–2771
15. Ma XY, Yin QS, Wu ZH, Xia H, Riew KD, Liu JF (2010) C2 anatomy and dimensions relative to translaminar screw placement in an Asian population. Spine 35(6):704–708
16. Wright NM (2004) Posterior C2 fixation using bilateral, crossing C2 laminar screws: case series and technical note. J Spinal Disord Tech 17:158–162
17. Yue B, Kwak DS, Kim MK, Kwon SO, Han SH (2010) Morphometric trajectory analysis for the C2 crossing laminar screw technique. Eur Spine J 19(5):828–832
18. Wang MY (2006) C2 crossing laminar screws: cadaveric morphometric analysis. Neurosurgery 59(1 Suppl 1):59, ONS-84-88
19. Heggeness M, Doherty B (1993) The trabecular anatomy of the axis. Spine 18:1945–1949
20. Korres DS, Karachalios TH, Roidis N, Lycomitros V et al (2004) Structural properties of the axis studied in cadaveric specimens. Cin Ortop Rel Res 418:134–140
21. Panjabi M, Duranceau J, Goel V et al (1991) Cervical human vertebrae. Quantitative three-dimensional anatomy for the middle and lower regions. Spine 16(8):861–869
22. Steinmetz MP, Mroz TE, Benzel EC (2010) Craniovertebral junction: biomechanical considerations. Neurosurgery 66(3 Suppl):7–12
23. Menezes AH, Traynelis VC (2008) Anatomy and biomechanics of normal cranio-vertebral junction and biomechanics of stabilization. Childs Nerv Syst 24:1091–1100
24. Panjabi M, Dvorak J, Crisco J III, Oda T, Hilibrand A, Grob D (1991) Flexion, extension, and lateral bending of the upper cervical spine in response to alar ligament transections. J Spinal Disord 4:157–167
25. Tubbs RS, Hallock JD, Radcliff V et al (2011) Ligaments of the craniocervical junction. A review. J Neurosurg Spine 14:697–709
26. Tsakotos GA, Anagnostopoulou SI, Evangelopoulos DS, Vasilopoulou M, Kontovazenitis PI, Korres SD (2007) Arnold's ligament and its contribution to the neck–tongue syndrome (NTS). Eur J Orthop Surg Traumatol 17:527–531
27. Fielding JW, Cochran GB, Lawsing JF III, Hohl M (1974) Tears of the transverse ligament of the atlas. A clinical and biomechanical study. J Bone Joint Surg Am 56:1683–1691
28. Haffajee MR, Thompson C, Govender S (2008) The supraodontoid space or "apical cave" at the craniocervical junction: a microdissection study. Clin Anat 21:405–415
29. Tubbs RS, Grabb P, Spooner A, Wilson W, Oakes WJ (2000) The apical ligament: anatomy and functional significance. J Neurosurg 92(2 Suppl):197–200
30. Dvorak J, Panjabi M (1987) Functional anatomy of the alar ligaments. Spine 12:183–189
31. Baumert B, Wörtler K, Steffinger D, Schmidt GP, Reiser MF, Baur-Melnyk A (2009) Assessment of the internal craniocervical ligaments with a new magnetic resonance imaging sequence: three-dimensional turbo spin echo with variable flip-angle distribution (SPACE). Magn Reson Imaging 27(7):954–960
32. Tubbs RS, Mortazavi MM, Louis RG, Loukas M, Shoja MM, Chern JJ, Benninger B, Cohen-Gadol AA (2012) The anterior atlantodental ligament: its anatomy and potential functional significance. World Neurosurg 77(5–6):775–777
33. Tubbs RS, Griessenauer CJ, McDaniel JG, Burns AM, Kumbla A, Cohen-Gadol AA (2010) The transverse occipital ligament: anatomy and potential

functional significance. Neurosurgery 66(3 Suppl Operative):1–3

34. Dvorak J, Schneider E, Saldinger P, Rahn B (1988) Biomechanics of the craniocervical region: the alar and transverse ligaments. J Orthop Res 6:452–461

35. Lang J (1986) Craniocervical region, osteology, and articulations. Neuro-Orthopedics 1:67–92

36. Tubbs RS, Dixon J, Loukas M, Shoja MM, Cohen-Gadol AA (2010) Ligament of Barkow of the craniocervical junction: its anatomy and potential clinical and functional significance. J Neurosurg Spine 12:619–622

37. Lang J, Kessler B (1991) About the suboccipital part of the vertebral artery and the neighboring bone-joint and nerve relationships. Skull Base Surg 1(1):64–72

38. Tubbs RS, Loukas M, Yalçin B, Shoja MM, Cohen-Gadol AA (2009) Classification and clinical anatomy of the first spinal nerve: surgical implications. J Neurosurg Spine 10(4):390–394

39. Sherk HH, Parke WW (1983) Normal adult anatomy. In: Bailey RW, Sherk HH et al (eds) The cervical spine. JB Lippincott, pp 8–22

40. Sato K, Watanabe T, Yoshimoto T, Kameyama M (1994) Magnetic resonance imaging of C2 segmental type of vertebral artery. Surg Neurol 41:45–51

41. Yamazaki M, Koda M, Aramomi MA, Hashimoto M, Masaki Y, Okawa A (2005) Anomalous vertebral artery at the extraosseous and intraosseous regions of the craniovertebral junction: analysis by three-dimensional computed tomography angiography. Spine (Phila Pa 1976) 30(21):2452–2457

42. Haffajee MR (1997) A contribution by the ascending pharyngeal artery to the arterial supply of the odontoid process of the axis vertebra. Clin Anat 10(1):14–18

43. Schiff DCM, Parke WW (1973) The arterial supply of the odontoid process. J Bone Joint Surg Am 55-A:1450–1456

Biomechanics

3

Vassilis A. Lykomitros

The human cervical spine has a unique anatomy adapted to accommodate the needs and stability of the highly mobile head–torso transition area. This is achieved through the presence of the upper cervical spine that includes the occipito-atlantal (C0–C1) and the atlantoaxial (C1–C2) joint complexes [1]. The internal architecture of the axis has also been studied by many authors [2, 3] and plays an important role to upper spinal stability.

White and Panjabi [4] defined clinical stability as the ability of the spine under physiologic loads to maintain its pattern of displacement so that there is no initial or additional neurologic deficit, no major deformity and no incapacitating pain. They further defined physiologic loads as loads that are incurred during normal activity. These definitions have been most useful when evaluating afflictions of the cervical spine, be it from trauma, degenerative conditions, tumors, or surgery. Atlantoaxial instability (AAI) is characterized by excessive movement at the junction between the atlas and axis as a result of either a bony or a ligamentous abnormality [4, 5].

The atlantoaxial (C1–C2) complex is composed of two facet joints and the unique atlantodental articulation. Stability at this highly mobile area primarily depends on ligamentous structures. Flexion and extension (sagittal plane) motion has been reported by several authors to be on average 11° and may be facilitated by a rounded tip of the dens. Rotation in the upper cervical spine represents 60 % of the entire cervical spine rotation and has been reported to be between 39° and 47° on each side. Lateral bending is minimal [6] (Figs. 3.1 and 3.2).

The instantaneous axis of rotation (IAR) for sagittal plane motion is located in the region of the middle third of the odontoid process, and for axial rotation it is located in the central axis of the odontoid process. Posterior translation is prevented by mechanical abutment of the anterior portion of the atlas on the odontoid process. Anterior translation is prevented primarily by the transverse ligament. The paired alar ligaments, through their anterior atlantodental component, provide secondary restraint. The accessory atlantoaxial ligaments and capsular ligaments are tertiary stabilizers. Anterior atlantoaxial subluxation increases the predental space. Up to 3 mm of anterior translation of the atlas on the axis, as measured at the anterior atlantodental interval (AADI), is normal. If this interval is increased, the transverse ligament must be attenuated, and if passes 6 mm or more, the transverse ligament and accessory stabilizing ligaments have been ruptured. The transverse ligament also protects the atlantoaxial joint from a rotatory dislocation . With the transverse ligament intact, a complete bilateral dislocation can occur at 65° of rotation. With transverse

V. A. Lykomitros (✉)
Hippokration General Hospital, 4 Filikis Eterias,
Panorama, Thessaloniki 55236, Greece
e-mail: vlikom@hotmail.com

D. S. Korres (ed.), *The Axis Vertebra*,
DOI: 10.1007/978-88-470-5232-1_3, © Springer-Verlag Italia 2013

Fig. 3.1 Neutral zone

	C0–C1	C1–C2	C2–C3
Flexion	3.3 ± 1.8	4.6 ± 2.4	0.7 ± 0.6
Extension	13.9 ± 4.1	8.7 ± 6.7	1.0 ± 0.7
Axial rotation	2.5 ± 1.6	39.6 ± 7.5	1.1 ± 0.5
Lateral bending	3.6 ± 1.5	2.4 ± 1.2	4.1 ± 1.1

Fig. 3.2 Range of motion

	C0–C1	C1–C2	C2–C3
Flexion	7.2 ± 2.5	12.3 ± 2.0	3.5 ± 1.3
Extension	20.2 ± 4.6	12.1 ± 6.5	2.7 ± 1.0
Axial rotation	9.9 ± 3.0	56.7 ± 4.8	3.3 ± 0.8
Lateral bending	9.1 ± 1.5	6.5 ± 2.3	9.6 ± 1.8

ligament rupture, dislocation can occur at 45° of rotation. Finally, the paired alar ligaments also restrict rotatory motion, since sectioning of one ligament will increase contralateral rotation [1].

Useful for determination of transverse ligament integrity is the rule of Spence [7] that states that if the amount of overhang of the lateral mass of the atlas on the lateral mass of the axis is greater than 6.9 mm, then the transverse ligament is probably torn [8]. Atlantoaxial instability is more common than occipito-cervical and can be the result of trauma, upper respiratory infection, rheumatoid arthritis or tumor, congenital anomalies, syndromes, or metabolic diseases [8].

Patients with atlantoaxial subluxation have sigmoid pattern in their time-displacement curves in sagittal rotation [9]. In these cases, atlantoaxial motion shows different points of the onset of rapid increase in motion in their sigmoid curves between flexion and extension. In most of the patients with atlantoaxial instability, subluxation occurred when the atlantoaxial joints were still in a more extended position and they were reduced when they were still in more flexed position.

A V-shaped predental space is not indicative of instability and can measure 0–18°, with a mean value of 6° in neutral and 9° in flexion [10]. In traumatic cases where a V-shaped predental space is discovered, it is possible that the transverse ligament may be attenuated and the anterior ring of the atlas hinges on the anterior atlantodental ligaments, as described by Dvorak and Panjabi [4, 11].

Sagittal plane axial instability is indicative of an underlying pathologic process. Compressive loads are transferred to the lateral mass articulation of the C1–C2 joints. Fractures of the atlas ring with disruption of the transverse ligament or erosive destruction can result in basilar invagination. Total lateral displacement of >6.9 mm of the lateral masses of the atlas over the masses of the axis as measured in an anteroposterior radiograph is indicative of a burst fracture of the atlas with insufficiency of the transverse ligament. Clinical stability at the occipito-cervical and atlantoaxial joints is intimately linked through their functional anatomy [12].

There are several disease processes and common injuries that tend to affect the ligaments of the craniocervical junction. The prevalence of atlantoaxial instability in children with Down syndrome is estimated to be between 9 and 30 %. This instability is thought to be due to ligamentous laxity as well as osseous structural abnormalities at the craniocervical junction [8, 12]. Odontoid fractures produced a slightly larger increase in atlantoaxial angular range of motion than ligament disruptions but a smaller increase in occipito-cervical range of motion. The different injuries affect the neutral zone and the position of atlantoaxial axis of rotation differently [13].

3.1 Biomechanics of the Craniocervical Junction

The combination of the bony anatomy, joint orientations and articulations, and ligamentous attachments of the craniovertebral junction allows rotation, flexion, extension, and, to a lesser extent, lateral bending. The atlantoaxial joints allow motion in flexion, extension, axial rotation, and lateral bending, owing to the biconvex and inherently unstable structure of the joint [1]. The occipito-atlantoaxial complex functions as a single unit that facilitates movement of the head about the spine. A unique aspect of this area is that the segmental structures between the occiput and the atlas and between the atlas and axis do not provide any significant stability. The loose joint capsules and the thin atlantoaxial and atlantooccipital membranes tolerate an extensive range of motion but impart minimal stability. Rather, stability in the occipito-atlantoaxial region is provided by the internal ligaments and muscles directly between the occiput and the axis.

The occipito-atlantoaxial region is particularly vulnerable to injury in children younger than 10 years of age [12]. The relatively large head and shorter neck of the young child places the fulcrum of the cervical spine within the occipito-atlantoaxial complex. Impact involving either the head or the torso can accelerate the head relative to the torso to concentrate the disruptive forces in the occipito-atlantoaxial region. The occipito-atlantoaxial complex is also inherently more unstable in this age group with more pliant ligaments, underdeveloped musculature, smaller condyles, and horizontal joint orientations. As a result, occipito-atlantoaxial injuries in children are mostly ligamentous in nature [8].

The pediatric atlantooccipital joint permits 10° of flexion and 25° of extension. The adult atlantooccipital joint provides approximately 15° of flexion and extension. The remaining flexion and extension of the cervical region comes from the vertebral segments below. Overall, the range of motion throughout the cervical region is greater in children than in late adolescents or adults. In children up to 10 years of age, the flexion and extension are centered around C2–C3, but this moves down to C4–C5 and C5–C6 after the age of 10 years. The axis normally moves forward on the C3, up to 2–3 mm in pediatric patients. When the head is flexed, this displacement is expected and can be exaggerated in the presence of muscle spasm. This pseudosubluxation does not represent instability, even though significant angulation may be present [8, 12]. The craniocervical junction is composed of 2 major joints: the atlantooccipital and the atlantoaxial joints. These joints are responsible for the majority of the movement of the cervical spine and operate on different biomechanical principles. The mechanical properties of the atlantooccipital joint are primarily determined by bony structures, whereas the mechanical properties of the atlantoaxial joint are mainly determined by ligamentous structures. The prominent movements at the atlantooccipital joint are flexion and extension. The various movements at this joint occur because the condyles glide in the sockets of the atlas. Panjabi et al. [4, 12] found the atlantooccipital joint to be responsible for 27.1° of flexion and 24.9° of extension. They also noted that about 8° of axial rotation can take place at this joint as well as minimal lateral and axial rotation and anteroposterior translation. Similar values are reported in the literature, with a mean movement of 23–24.5° of flexion/extension, whereas axial rotation was limited to 2.4–7.2° [12]. Flexion is limited by impingement of the odontoid process on the foramen magnum, and extension is restricted by the tectorial membrane. Lateral flexion is strongly inhibited at the atlantooccipital joint by the contralateral alar ligament. The primary movement at the atlantoaxial joint is axial rotation. Steinmetz et al. [9] reported that the mean axial rotational movement was between 23.3 and 38.9°. Flexion and extension at the atlantoaxial joint range from 10.1 to 22.4° and are limited by the transverse ligament and tectorial membrane, respectively. Lateral bending is restricted to 6.7°

by the contralateral alar ligament, and some very minimal anteroposterior translation may occur at this joint. Although these 2 joints function differently, they must act in unison to ensure optimal stability and mobility at the craniocervical junction.

There is a wide range of atlantoaxial rotation in normal subjects. At the extremes of physiologic rotation in healthy subjects, there is striking but incomplete loss of contact between the articular surfaces of the atlas and the axis. The range of rotation to the right was 20–48.5° (mean, 32.4°) and to the left was 13–52.75° (mean, 34.2°). There was no significant difference between rotation to the right and left. Total rotation was 45–88.5° (mean, 69.25°). The appearances of the rotated atlantoaxial joint are striking and may be misinterpreted as subluxation.

Lateral bending in the cervical region is generally accompanied by rotation resulting from the oblique orientation of the superior and inferior facets. During rightward rotation of the axis on the atlas, the left transverse foramen of the atlas moves anteriorly, whereas the right transverse foramen moves posteriorly relative to the adjacent axis. As the rotation increases, the increased distance between adjacent transverse foramina results in increased tensile forces on the vertebral artery and spinal nerve.

3.2   Biomechanics of the Occipito-Atlantoaxial Ligaments

The transverse ligament is the major stabilizing ligament at the atlantoaxial joint. The atlantoaxial joint is responsible for about 47° of rotation at the neck. The transverse ligament permits rotation to occur, while the alar ligaments prevent excessive rotation and are most vulnerable to rupture under either rapid or slow loading forces. The biomechanical data reported by Fielding et al. [14] demonstrated that the transverse ligament is the primary defense against anterior subluxation of the atlas on the axis and that it is relatively inelastic, only allowing the axis to subluxate approximately 3–5 mm before

rupture. They also concluded that the accessory ligaments of the atlantoaxial joints (namely the alar ligaments) serve as secondary restrictions of the atlas to anterior shift [15].

The alar ligaments function as stabilizing structures of the atlantoaxial joint and act to limit axial rotation and lateral bending on the contralateral side. If the transverse ligament ruptures, the alar ligaments become responsible for preventing atlantal subluxation. Following the rupture of the transverse ligament, a mean force of 72 kg was needed to stretch the alar ligament to create a predental space of 12 mm, and any subluxation greater that 12 mm caused the alar ligament to rupture. The alar ligament limits axial rotation on the contralateral side to about 90°. Damage to this ligament results in further axial rotation, which can result in compression or damage to the vertebral artery or the spinal accessory nerves [15].

The transverse occipital ligament (TOL) is thought to have similar functions to the alar ligaments in helping to stabilize the craniocervical junction. Lang et al. [16] believed the TOL represented the uppermost fibers of the alar ligament that sometimes crossed the midline. However, Tubbs et al. [17] did not consistently find a connection between the TOL and the odontoid process or alar ligaments. When attached to the alar ligament, the possible functions of the TOL include providing additional support in stabilizing lateral bending, flexion, and axial rotation of the head [15].

Several authors believe that the accessory atlantoaxial ligament functions similarly to the alar ligament in maintaining stability at the craniocervical junction as well as limiting axial rotation of the head. Another possible function is protection and support for branches of the vertebral artery that supply the odontoid process. Dvorak et al. [11] suggested that this ligament, along with the alar ligament, tectorial membrane and joint capsule, functions to limit axial rotation of the head. Tubbs et al. [18] found that axial rotation of the head between 5 and 8° caused maximal tension in the contralateral accessory atlantoaxial ligament. The ligament also resisted flexion maximally between 5 and

10° and was lax in normal extension of the spine. The accessory atlantoaxial ligament coupled with the alar ligament maintained proper atlantal-axial-occipital alignment by forming a halter for the odontoid [15].

The lateral atlantooccipital (LAO) ligament plays a role in limiting lateral flexion of the head [19]. Lateral flexion of the head occurs almost exclusively in the subaxial spine, although Panjabi et al. [5, 6] reported that lateral flexion of the atlantooccipital joint may range from 8 to 40°. The mean tensile strength of 37.5 N is relatively substantial and indicates that this ligament may play a role in maintaining stability at the craniocervical junction. When the LAO ligament was transected in cadavers, Tubbs et al. [17] observed an increase in lateral flexion of the contralateral side of 3–5°. Additionally, the LAO ligament may play a small role in limiting axial rotation of the atlantooccipital joint. Tubbs et al. [19] noted tautness of the LAO ligament on contralateral rotation of the head on the atlas [15].

The apical ligament, anterior and posterior atlantooccipital membranes , and the tectorial membrane are crucial elements for providing craniocervical junction stability [20]. The apical ligament is lax, while the head is in the neutral position and no tautness can be produced following cranial distraction [15, 21].

The tectorial membrane restricts extension at the atlantooccipital joint and flexion/extension at the atlantoaxial joint. Oda et al. [22], however, found that this membrane restricts flexion between the occiput, atlas, and axis and has no limiting effect on extension. Some authors [15, 23, 24] have found that the tectorial membrane together with its lateral band (the Arnold ligament) plays a substantial role in maintaining stability at the craniocervical junction, especially in limiting flexion. They found [25] that flexion of the craniocervical junction made the tectorial membrane fully taut at 15°, and extension made the tectorial membrane fully taut at 20°. The tensile strength of this ligament was found to be 76 N. The tectorial membrane could not be made taut with any lateral flexion or axial rotation of the joint [15].

The nuchal ligament restricts hyperflexion of the cervical spine. Interestingly, some have identified a greater concentration of proprioceptive fibers in this structure and have opined that it may play a role in maintaining proper alignment of the cervical spine [15, 26].

The anterior atlantooccipital (AAO) and posterior atlantooccipital (PAO) membranes are grouped as soft tissue structures critical to maintaining stability of the cranio cervical junction (CCJ). The AAO membrane may function synergistically with the Barkow ligament to limit atlantooccipital extension of the head [15]. Actions of the cervical musculature, including the suboccipital musculature between the occiput and the axis, are also thought to play a significant role in securing the cranium firmly to the spine.

References

1. Ghanayem AJ et al., (2004) Functional anatomy of joints, ligaments, and discs. In Clark CR, Ducker TB, Benzel E, et al. (eds) The cervical spine. The cervical spine research society, 4th edn. Lippincott Williams & Wilkins, Philadelphia, pp 46–54
2. Korres DS, Karahalios TH, Roidis N, Lykomitros VA et al (2004) Structural properties of the axis studied in cadaveric specimens. Clin Orthop Related Res 418:134–140
3. Amling M, Post N, Wening VJ et al (1995) Structural heterogeneity within the axis: the main cause in the etiology of dens fractures: a histomorphometric analysis of 37 normal and osteoporotic autopsy cases. J Neurosurg 83:330–335
4. White AA, Panjabi MM (1990) Clinical biomechanics of the spine, 2nd edn. Lippincott JP, Philadelphia
5. Panjabi MM, Crisco JJ, Vasavada A et al (2001) Mechanical properties of the human cervical spine as shown by three-dimensional load-displacement curves. Spine 26(24):2692–2700
6. Panjabi M M et al (2004) Cervical spine kinematics and clinical instability. In Clark C R, Ducker T B, Benzel E et al (eds) The cervical spine. The cervical spine research society, 4th edn. Lippincott Williams & Wilkins, pp 57–77
7. Spence KF Jr, Decker S, Sell KW (1970) Bursting atlantal fracture associated with rupture of the transverse ligament. J Bone Joint Surg Am 52:543–549
8. Jagannathan J, Dumont AS, Prevedello DM et al (2007) Cervical spine injuries in pediatric athletes:

mechanisms and management. Neurosurg Focus 21(4):E6

9. Steinmetz MP, Mroz TE, Benzel EC (2010) Craniovertebral junction: biomechanical considerations. Neurosurgery 66:A7–A12

10. Morishita Y, Falakassa J, Naito M et al (2009) The kinematic relationships of the upper cervical spine. Spine 34(24):2642–2645

11. Dvorak J, Panjabi MM, Gerber M (1987) CT-functional diagnostics of the rotatory instability of the upper cervical spine: an experimental study in cadavers. Spine 12:197

12. Panjabi MM, Myers BS (2009) Cervical spine protection report. Prepared for NOCSAE. National Operating Committee on Standards for Athletic Equipment. http://nocsae.org/research/rep/SpineReport.pdf. Accessed 22 Dec

13. Crawford NR, Hurlbert JR, Choi WG, Dickman CA (1999) Differential biomechanical effects of injury and wiring at C1–C2. Spine 24(18):1894–1902

14. Fielding JW, Cochran GB, Lawsing JF III, Hohl M (1974) Tears of the transverse ligament of the atlas: a clinical and biomechanical study. J Bone Joint Surg Am 56:1683–1691

15. Tubbs RS, Hallock JD, Radcliff V, Naftel RP et al (2011) Ligaments of the craniocervical junction. A review. J Neurosurg Spine 14:697–709

16. Lang J (1995) Skull base and related structures. Schattauer, Stuttgart

17. Tubbs RS, Griessenauer CJ, McDaniel JG, Burns AM, Kubla A, Cohen-Gobel AA (2010) The transverse occipital ligament: anatomy and potential functional significance. Neurosurgery 66(3 Suppl Operative):1–3

18. Tubbs RS, Salter EG, Oakes WJ (2004) The accessory atlantoaxial ligament. Neurosurgery 55:400–402

19. Tubbs RS, Stetler W, Shoja MM, Loukas M, Hansasuta A, Liechty P et al (2007) The lateral atlantooccipital ligament. Surg Radiol Anat 29:219–223

20. Grab BC, Frye TA, Hedlund GL, Vaid YN, Grabb PA, Royal SA (1999) MRI diagnosis of suspected atlanto-occipital dissociation in childhood. Pediatr Radiol 29:275–281

21. Tubbs RS, Grabb P, Spooner A, Wilson W, Oakes WJ (2000) The apical ligament: anatomy and functional significance. J Neurosurg Spine 92:197–200

22. Oda T, Panjabi MM, Crisco JJ, Buef HU, Grob D, Dvorak J (1992) Role of the tectorial membrane in the stability of the upper cervical spine. Clin Biomech (Bristol, Avon) 7:201–207

23. Krakenes J, Kaale BR, Nordii H, Moen G, Rorvik J, Gilhus NE (2003) MR analysis of the transverse ligament in the late stage of whiplash injury. Acta Radiol 44:637–644

24. Tsakotos GA, Anagnostopoulou SI, Evangelopoulow DS et al (2007) The Arnol's ligament and its contribution to the neck-tongue syndrome (NTS). J Ortthop Surg Traumatolo 17:527–531

25. Tubbs RS, Kelly DR, Humphrey ER, Chua GD, Shoja MM, Salter EG et al (2007) The tectorial membrane: anatomical, biomechanical, and histological analysis. Clin Anat 20:382–386

26. Lang J (1986) Craniocervical region, osteology and articulations. Neuro-Orthopedics 1:67–92

Imaging

4

Konstantinos E. Kokkinis and Emmanouil Emmanouil

4.1 Radiography

The radiographic investigation of the axis is demanding and needs particular attention, since it is closely related to specific anatomic elements that are superimposed on each other interfering and confusing the radiographic views. The need for patient's cooperation is important. The involved anatomic elements should be evaluated with specific views.

The radiographic investigation of the axis should include the occipito-cervical complex with specific views including the antero-posterior oblique, the bilateral postero-anterior and the antero-posterior (open mouth) view. The atlantoaxial radiologic imaging should also include specific views to visualize the atlantoaxial joints and the odontoid process.

4.1.1 Lateral View

The patient: Supine; adjust the body in a true antero-posterior (AP) body position. The arms are along the sides of the body, and the shoulders are lying in the same transverse plane.

The cassette: Must be placed in the vertical position and in contact with the upper neck. Then, it is placed at the middle line, at the level of the atlantoaxial articulation (2.5 cm distal to the tip of the mastoid process). The position of the cassette must be parallel with the midsagittal plane of the neck (Fig. 4.1). The neck must be extended so that the shadow of the mandibular rami will not superimpose the spine. The head is positioned so that the midsagittal plane is perpendicular to the table. The patient must hold his breath.

Central ray: Must be perpendicularly to a point 2.5 cm distal to the mastoid tip.

Imaging: Shows the atlas and axis, and the atlantooccipital articulations (Fig. 4.2). Some authors [1] suggest that the head must be slightly rotated to prevent superimposition of the lamina of the atlas and recommend a slight transverse tilt of the head for better view of the arches of the atlas.

Pitfalls: The upper cervical vertebra should be included. The neck should be extended so that the rami of the mandible will not overlap the upper cervical spine, and the rami of the mandible should be nearly superimposed [2]. Some authors [3] slightly extend the patient's neck with the mouth wide open. The central ray is positioned at 35° caudal and to the middle line of the third cervical vertebra. The exposure is made with the head passively rotated 10° to the side, thus removing the mandible from the underlying areas of interest.

K. E. Kokkinis · E. Emmanouil (✉)
KAT Hospital, Nikis 2, 14561,
Kiffisia Athens, Greece
e-mail: emmanouilemmanouil@yahoo.gr

D. S. Korres (ed.), *The Axis Vertebra*,
DOI: 10.1007/978-88-470-5232-1_4, © Springer-Verlag Italia 2013

Fig. 4.1 Lateral atlas and axis

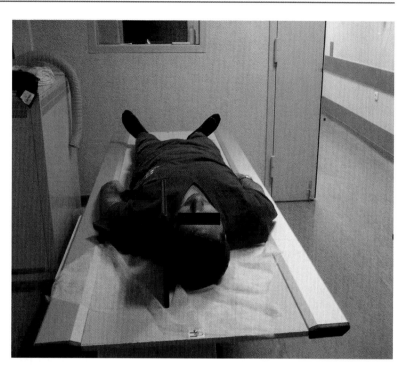

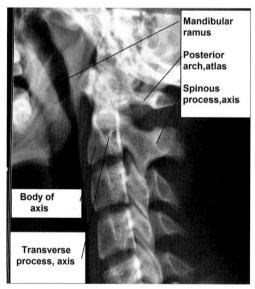

Fig. 4.2 Lateral view

4.1.2 AP View: Open Mouth

The open-mouth view was described by Albers-Schonberg [4] in 1910 and by George [5] in 1919.

The patient: Supine; the arms are along the sides of the body.

The cassette: At the level of the second cervical segment, to the middle line, in the Bucky tray. Patient's head must be placed so that the midsagittal plane is perpendicular to the plane of the table (Fig. 4.3). The patient must open his mouth as wide as possible, and the head is stabilized so that the line from the lower edge of the upper incisors to the tip of the mastoid process is perpendicular to the film. The patient should keep his mouth wide open and at the same time to say softly "ah" in order to keep his tongue in the floor of his mouth so that its shadow will not be projected on that of the atlas and axis. Mandible should be still.

Central ray: Perpendicular to the midpoint of the open mouth.

Imaging: Shows an AP projection of the atlas and axis through the open mouth (Fig. 4.4). In cases the patient has either a deep head or a long mandible, the atlas cannot be demonstrated.

Criteria: The odontoid process, atlas, axis and atlantoaxial articulations should be well demonstrated. The mouth should be wide open, and the shadow of the tongue should not be projected over the atlas and axis [2].

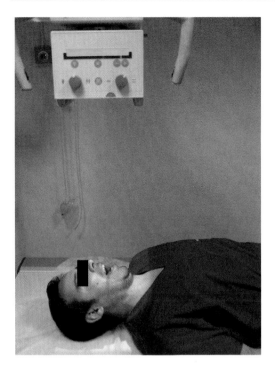

Fig. 4.3 AP atlas and axis

4.1.3 Odontoid Process

4.1.3.1 AP View: Fuchs Method

The patient: Supine; the arms are along the sides of the body.

The cassette: In the Bucky tray, to the middle line at the level of the tips of the mastoid processes. Chin extended; chin and tip of the mastoid process are vertical. We stabilize the head so that the midsagittal plane is perpendicular to the plane of the table. The patient must hold his breath (Fig. 4.5).

Central ray: Perpendicular to the midpoint of the film; it enters the neck distal to the tip of the chin.

Imaging: Shows an AP view of the odontoid process lying within the shadow of the foramen magnum (Fig. 4.6). Fuchs [6] described this view for the odontoid process in case that its upper half is not clearly shown in the open-mouth view. It is useful in cases of suspected fractures or degenerative disease of the upper cervical spine.

Criteria: The entire odontoid process should be seen through the foramen magnum without any rotation of the head or neck [2].

4.1.3.2 PA View: Judd Method

The patient: Prone; the elbows are flexed and the shoulders in the same transverse plane.

The cassette: The patient must extend his neck and rest his chin on the table. The Bucky tray is positioned so that the midpoint is entered into the throat at the level of the upper margin of

Fig. 4.4 Open-mouth view

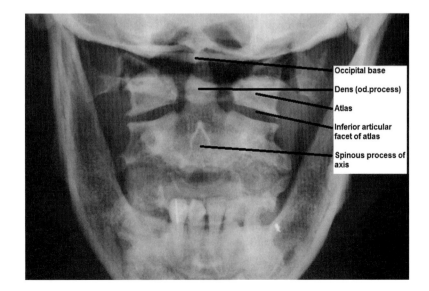

Occipital base

Dens (od.process)

Atlas

Inferior articular facet of atlas

Spinous process of axis

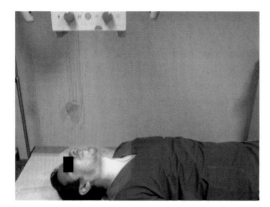

Fig. 4.5 AP odontoid process

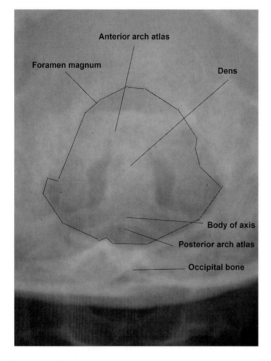

Anterior arch atlas

Foramen magnum

Dens

Body of axis

Posterior arch atlas

Occipital bone

Fig. 4.6 AP view

the thyroid cartilage (Fig. 4.7). The tip of the nose must be approximately 2.5 cm from the table top (approximately 37° to the plane of the film). The midsagittal plane must be perpendicular to the table. The patient must hold his breath.

Central ray: Perpendicular to the midpoint of the film. It enters the occiput just posterior to the mastoid tips. Should not be used in case of

degenerative disease or suspected fractures of the upper cervical spine.

Imaging: Shows a PA projection of the odontoid process through the foramen magnum (Fig. 4.6b).

Criteria: The entire dens should be seen through the foramen magnum without any rotation of the head or neck [2].

4.1.3.3 AP Axial Oblique View: Kasabach Method

The patient: Supine; the arms are along the sides of the body.

The cassette: In the Bucky tray, to the middle line of the midsagittal plane at the level of the mastoid tip. The head must be rotated approximately 40–45° opposite to the side being examined. The infraorbitomeatal line must be perpendicular to the plane of the table. The patient must hold his breath (Fig. 4.8). In case of right-angle projections of the dens we can perform one exposure with the head turned to the right and one with the head turned to the left.

Central ray: In 10–15° caudal to the middle line, midway between the outer canthus and the external auditory meatus.

Imaging: Kasabach [7] presented this technique for use in conjunction with the AP and lateral (Fig. 4.9). In case of a possible fracture or degenerative disease, the head should not be rotated. Kasabach suggested rotation of the body rather than only the head.

Criteria: The odontoid process should be clearly seen. Some authors [8] described a position to demonstrate the atlantooccipital–odontoid process relationship; the central ray is directed vertically midway between the mastoid processes at the level of the occipito-cervical joints [2].

4.2   Computed Tomography

Computed tomography (CT) is frequently employed for the evaluation of the spine; helical and multislice techniques have been introduced. After placing the neck in the isocenter of gantry,

Fig. 4.7 PA odontoid
process

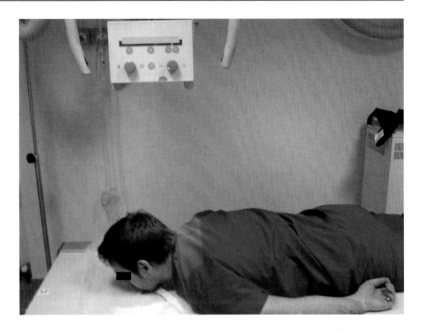

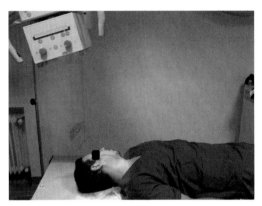

Fig. 4.8 AP axial oblique view

axial sections are adjusted to the plane of atlas
and axis. Basic evaluation can be performed by
axial scanning at 0° of angulation. Scanning of
the whole region is easy and has the advantage
that reformations can be adjusted in every plane.
With multislice CT, for the highest possible
resolution in the cervical spine, section colli-
mation may be reduced to 0.5–0.75 mm. This
will generate an almost isotropic data set that
enables the highest quality multiplanar refor-
mation (MPR) in any direction. MPR views are
tailored to the specific problem, and most
orthopedic and trauma cases will require

evaluation on a second plane (coronal, sagittal).
MPR requires prior reconstruction of an over-
lapping thin-section data set (secondary row data
set). Image reconstruction uses a small field of
view to ensure optimum spatial resolution.
Three-dimensional images (3D) are useful in
patients with complex fractures and obscure
findings and anatomic details. For 3D CT, a
volume-rendering technique (VRT) is preferred,
but shaded-surface displays (SSDs) are also
possible (Figs. 4.10, 4.11). Image reconstruction
uses a small field of view to ensure optimum
spatial resolution. In trauma patients, reconstruction with a high-resolution (bone) algorithm
is normally used, but additional reconstructions
with a standard algorithm are needed for the
evaluation of the paraspinal soft tissues [9].

Some studies are performed with intravenous
contrast enhancement because of the increased
anatomic detail compared with noncontrast CT
[10]. Intrathecal contrast is used when precise
definition of the cord is necessary. It is also
helpful to better define the extent and degree of
subarachnoid space. Nonionic contrast material
is administered via C1–C2 injection, followed
by myelographic filming and immediate post-
myelogram focused CT scanning.

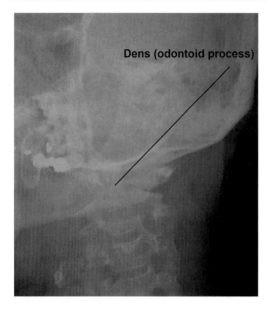

Fig. 4.9 AP axial oblique view

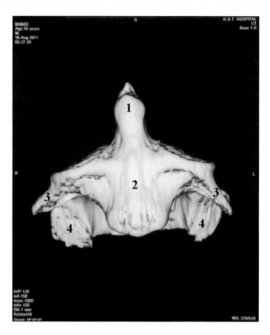

Fig. 4.11 CT 3D (VRT) image of the axis. Anterior view. Odontoid (*1*), body (*2*), transverse processes (*3*), inferior articular processes of the axis (*4*)

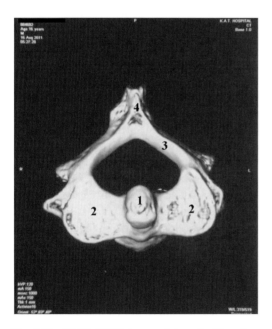

Fig. 4.10 CT 3D (VRT) image of the axis. View from head. Odontoid (*1*), superior facets (*2*), lamina (*3*), spinous process (*4*)

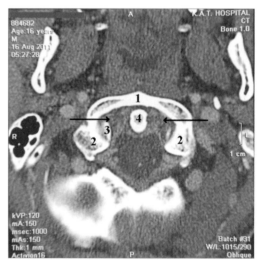

Fig. 4.12 An axial contrast-enhanced CT at the C1 level demonstrates the anterior arch of the atlas (*1*), the superior articulating facets (*2*), the occipital condyles (*3*), the odontoid (*4*) and the alar ligaments as they extend from the odontoid to the occipital condyles (*arrows*)

When scanning the craniocervical junction in a craniocaudal direction, the basiocciput is the first osseous structure imaged. The atlas is next visualized as scanning continues inferiorly (Figs. 4.12, 4.13, 4.14). Coronal imaging

demonstrates the craniocaudal slope of the atlantooccipital articulation from lateral to medial margins contributing to the lateral

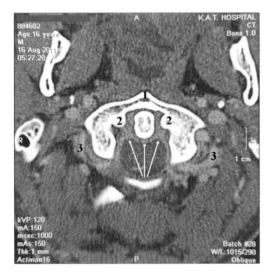

Fig. 4.13 A scan inferiorly shows the anterior tubercle of C1 (1), tubercles of the lateral masses of C1 (2), the vertebral arteries (3) and the transverse ligament and tectorial membrane with dura (arrows)

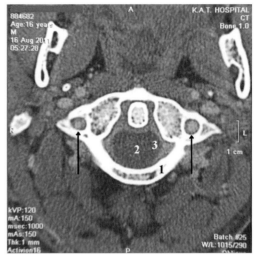

Fig. 4.14 A scan inferiorly demonstrates the posterior arch of the atlas (1), spinal cord (2), subarachnoid space containing CSF (3). The vertebral arteries as they pass through the foramina transversaria (arrows)

stability of the joint. The atlas is recognized as a ring formed by fused anterior and posterior arches. On 0° images, the anterior arch will frequently be imaged cephalad to posterior arch [11]. As scanning continues caudally, the inferior articular facets of the atlas are demonstrated. These appear circular in the axial plane and flat or slightly concave in the coronal plane. The inferior facets slope craniocaudally medially to laterally to articulate with the superior facets of the axis. This articulation permits a sliding motion to occur during head rotation.

The axis consists of a large body that is fused to the odontoid process, a superiorly projecting tubercle that extends from the body of the axis through the anterior third of the atlas ring (Figs. 4.15, 4.16, 4.17). The small transverse processes of the axis contain foramina transversaria for the vertebral arteries and veins. The spinal canal is large, but smaller than that of the atlas. The spinous process of the axis is massive and usually bifid [12].

The posterior longitudinal ligament is demonstrated dorsal to the body of the axis as a broad soft-tissue density measuring approximately 1 mm in thickness. The ligament is contiguous superiorly with the tectorial membrane, which

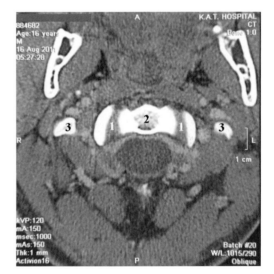

Fig. 4.15 An image at the base of the dens (2) demonstrates the atlantoaxial joints (1) and transverse processes of the atlas (3)

extends to the occiput. The tectorial membrane is imaged axially together with the closely approximated anterior dura as an enhancing soft-tissue density posterior to the odontoid process, which is contained between the lateral masses of the atlas (Fig. 4.18). The cruciate ligament is anterior to the tectorial membrane and

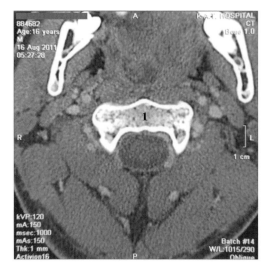

Fig. 4.16 A scan at the C2 body level (*1*)

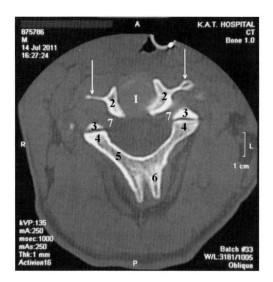

Fig. 4.17 At the C2–C3 level, the intervertebral disk is demonstrated (*1*), laterally the C3 uncinate processes are present (*2*), the superior articular processes of C3 are anterior (*3*), whereas the inferior articular processes of the axis are posterior (*4*), C2 lamina (*5*), C2 bifid spinous process (*6*). The facet joints make up the posterior and lateral aspect of the intervertebral foramina (*7*). C3 transverse processes (*arrows*)

contiguous with the posterior margin of the odontoid. This T-shaped ligament extends from the odontoid to the occiput (long axis) and between small medially facing tubercles that project from the lateral masses of the atlas (thick axis or transverse ligament). The transverse

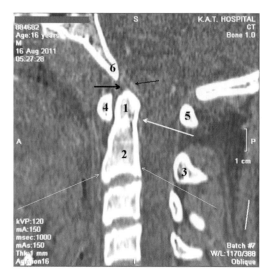

Fig. 4.18 CT sagittal MPR image. Odontoid (*1*), C2 body (*2*), C2 spinous process (*3*), anterior arch of C1 (*4*), posterior arch of C1 (*5*), basion (*6*). Apical ligament (*thick black arrow*). Tectorial membrane (*thin black arrow*). Transverse ligament (*thick white arrow*). Anterior and posterior longitudinal ligaments (*thin white arrows*)

ligament can occasionally be identified on axial images as an enhancing curvilinear soft-tissue density of variable thickness that is adjacent to the dorsal margin of the odontoid process (Fig. 4.13). The alar ligaments extend from the odontoid process to the medial inferior aspects of the occipital condyles. These ligaments may at times be seen on axial or coronal CT scans near the apex of the odontoid process as small paramedian soft-tissue densities separated by epidural fat (Fig. 4.19). Also, occasionally identified on coronal CT is the thin apical ligament that extends from the apex of the odontoid to the anterior rim of the foramen magnum [13].

The patulous subarachnoid space containing cerebrospinal fluid (CSF) generally provides adequate natural contrast for visualization of the spinal cord (Fig. 4.14). However, if detailed analysis of neural structures at this level is difficult, intrathecal contrast provides the necessary background for accurate CT evaluation. The cervical cord, nearly circular on axial images at the atlas level, gradually flattens through the mid-cervical levels and then again becomes nearly circular at the cervicothoracic junction. The

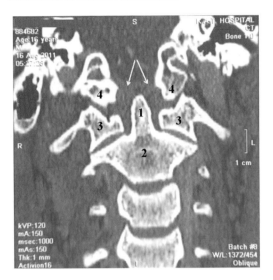

Fig. 4.19 CT coronal MPR image. Odontoid (*1*), C2 body (*2*), C1 lateral masses (*3*), the occipital condyles (*4*) are inferiorly convex protuberances that provide the articular surfaces for the concave *upper* aspect of the superior articular facets of the atlas. The inferior articular facets of the atlas are flat or slightly concave, and they slope craniocaudally to articulate with the superior facets of the axis. Alar ligaments (*arrows*)

position of the cord at the craniocervical junction is slightly anterior within the canal. The cord has homogenous appearance, with slightly indentations noted anteriorly and posteriorly representing the anterior and posterior median fissures [14].

4.3 Magnetic Resonance Imaging

The upper cervical spine has been extensively investigated by magnetic resonance imaging (MRI) as the method of choice for evaluation of many disease processes in the spine. Such evaluation focuses predominantly in the musculoskeletal (vertebral bodies, intervertebral foramina, ligaments and joints) and the nervous system (spinal cord and the exiting spinal nerve roots). Sagittal T1-weighted (T1W) and T2-weighted (T2W) sequences are a basic starting point for most examinations of the cervical spine, performed with conventional spin-echo (SE) technique or preferably with fast spin-echo (FSE) technique [15]. For T2W imaging FSE, MRI has almost completely replaced SE MRI.

The advantages of FSE T2W MRI are the shorter examination time and the better visualization of the spinal cord. The slice thickness should be no more than 3–4 mm, and the interslice gap should be no greater than 1 mm. A frequently selective fat saturation pulse can be applied with the T2W FSE sequence, or an FSE short-inversion-time inversion-recovery (STIR) sequence can be also used. To evaluate the upper cervical spine, an axial sequence is also needed. Axial gradient-echo (GRE) sequences have been found to provide a better depiction of the cervical neural foramina and the structures in the foramina than SE images. Two-dimensional (2D) Fourier transform GRE or 3D Fourier transform GRE sequences can be used. The 3D GRE technique is superior to the 2D GRE technique because it can provide thinner sections while maintaining good signal-to-noise and contrast. Coronal T1W or T2W images provide a unique look of the articulations of the upper cervical spine [16, 17].

The central sagittal image (Fig. 4.20) shows the full height of the odontoid. The spinous process of the axis and the atlantodental interval is almost completely seen. The basion is positioned above a small amount of adipose tissue that is normally seen between it and the odontoid process. The spinal cord is present in the spinal canal, surrounded by hyperintense CSF. Posterior to the odontoid process, an area of decreased signal intensity can be seen that represents the transverse ligament. The transverse ligament is better imaged in the axial plane. The transverse ligament arches across the ring of the atlas and retains the odontoid process in contact with the anterior arch of the atlas. A small fascicle extends upward and another extends downward from the transverse ligament as it crosses the odontoid process. The upper fasciculus attaches to the basilar portion of the occipital bone, and the lower fasciculus is fixed to the posterior surface of the body of the axis. This entire ligament is named the cruciate ligament of the atlas.

The ligamentum flavum connects the lamina of adjacent vertebrae and shows a hypointense band just posterior to the dura. Because of its elasticity, the ligamentum flavum helps preserve

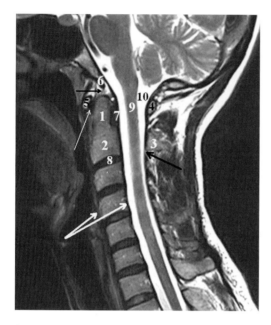

Fig. 4.20 MRI sagittal T2W FSE image. Odontoid (*1*), C2 body (*2*), C2 spinous process (*3*), posterior arch of C1 (*4*), anterior arch of C1 (*5*), basion (*6*), transverse ligament (*7*), C2–C3 intervertebral disk (*8*), spinal cord (*9*), CSF (*10*). Apical ligament (*thin black arrow*). Ligamentum flavum (*thick black arrow*). Atlantodental interval (*thin white arrow*). Anterior and posterior longitudinal ligaments (*thick white arrows*)

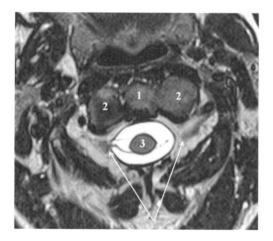

Fig. 4.21 MRI axial T2W 3D GRE image. Odontoid (*1*), anterior tubercle of C1 (*2*), *right* occipital condyle (*3*), spinal cord (*4*). Alar ligaments (*thin white arrows*). Dura (*thick white arrow*). Vertebral arteries (*black arrows*)

upright posture. The posterior atlantoaxial ligament replaces the ligamentum flavum between the atlas and axis. The anterior and posterior longitudinal ligaments are intimately adherent to the intervertebral disks and the vertebral margins. The longitudinal ligaments are not adherent to the middle of the vertebral bodies. The actual visualization of the anterior and posterior ligaments can be limited on MRI because of partial volume averaging with the adjacent vertebral body cortex.

The anterior aspect of the intervertebral disks is hypointense on the T2W and T1W images, representing the outer ring of the annulus fibrosus. The same signal intensity is also seen at the posterior aspect of the intervertebral disks, but is less distinct because the annulus fibrosus is thicker anteriorly than posteriorly. The disk endplates are well visualized as hypointense lines on the T2W and T1W images.

The axial T2W image through the top of the odontoid process shows a portion of the alar ligament. The alar ligament attaches to the top of the odontoid process and inserts to the medial aspect of the occipital condyles. The transverse ligament is present posterior to the odontoid process, attaching to the ring of the atlas. Anterior and posterior synovial joints make up the median atlantoaxial joint. The former is between the anterior arch of the atlas and the odontoid process, and the latter is between the odontoid process and the transverse ligament. On either side of the odontoid process are the lateral atlantoaxial joints, which are gliding joints (Fig. 4.21).

The vertebral arteries can be seen as they pass through the dura. The vertebral arteries pass beneath the posterior atlantooccipital membrane before entering the thecal sac. The dorsal root ganglia can be seen (Fig. 4.22). The gray matter can be faintly seen in the spinal cord. At the C2–C3 level, the intervertebral disk can be delineated, and laterally the C3 uncinate process is present. The vertebral artery is adjacent to the uncinate process (Figs. 4.23, 4.24). The CSF is dark on the T1W images, and the CSF-to-cord contrast is good. The neural foramina and visualization of the disks are not optimum on T1W images as on T2W images (Fig. 4.24).

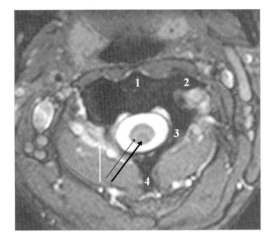

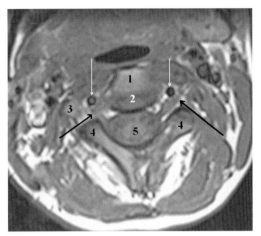

Fig. 4.22 MRI axial T2W GRE image. C2 body (*1*), C2 *left* transverse processes (*2*), C2 lamina (*3*), C2 spinous process (*4*). *White* marrow of the spinal cord (*thick black arrow*). Gray matter of the spinal cord (*thin black arrow*). Exiting right C2 spinal nerve root (*white arrow*)

Fig. 4.24 MRI axial T1W FSE image. C2 body (*1*), C2–C3 intervertebral disk (*2*), *right* transverse process of the axis (*3*), inferior articular processes of the axis (*4*), spinal cord (*5*). C3 spinal nerve roots (*black arrows*). Vertebral arteries (*white arrows*)

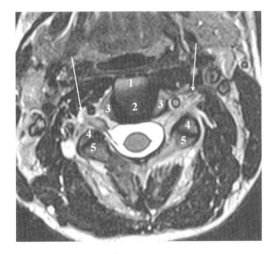

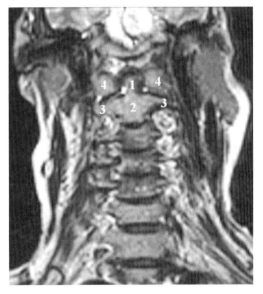

Fig. 4.23 MRI axial T2W 3D GRE image. C2 body (*1*), C2–C3 intervertebral disk (*2*), C3 uncinate processes (*3*), the superior articular processes of C3 are anterior (*4*), the inferior articular processes of the axis are posterior (*5*). C3 spinal nerve roots (*white arrows*)

Fig. 4.25 MRI coronal T2W FSE image. Odontoid (*1*), C2 body (*2*), C2 transverse processes (*3*), lateral masses of the atlas (*4*)

Coronal images provide a unique view of the articulations of cervical spine (Figs. 4.25, 4.26). The atlantooccipital joints, the lateral atlantoaxial joints, the intervertebral disks and the uncinate process are well shown. The alar ligament connecting the odontoid process to the occipital condyles is shown. The transverse ligament is not readily identified. Laterally the vertebral arteries ascend through the transverse foramina. Asymmetry of alar ligaments, craniocervical junction and C1–C2 facet joints and joint effusions are common in asymptomatic individuals. The clinical relevance of these MRI findings is therefore

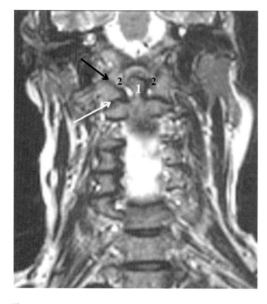

Fig. 4.26 MRI coronal T2W FSE image. Odontoid (*1*) and alar ligaments (*2*). *Right* atlantooccipital joint (*black arrow*). *Right* atlantoaxial joint (*white arrow*)

limited in the identification of the source of neck pain in symptomatic patients [18].

References

1. Pancoast HK, Pendergrass EP, Schaeffer JP (1940) The head and neck in roentgen diagnosis. Charles C Thomas Publisher, Springfield III
2. Ballinger PW (1991) Merrill's atlas of radiographic positions and radiologic procedures. School of Allied Medical Professions, The Ohio State University, Columbus
3. Smith G, Abel M (1975) Visualization of the posterolateral elements of the upper cervical vertebrae in the anteroposterior projection. Radiology 115:219–220
4. Albers-Schonberg HE (1910) Die Rontgentechnich, 3rd edn. Grafe&Sillem, Hamburg
5. George AW (1919) Method for more accurate study of injuries to the atlas and axis. Boston Med Surg J 181:395–398
6. Fuchs AW (1940) Cervical vertebrae (part1). Radiogr Clin Photogr 16:2–17
7. Kasabach HH (1939) A roentgenographic method for the study of the second cervical vertebrae. AJR 42:782–785
8. Hermann E, Stender H (1962) Ein einfache Aufnahmetechnik zur Darstellung der Dens axis. Forstschr Roentgenstr 96:115–119
9. Prokop M, Galanski M (2003) Spiral and multislice computed tomography of the body. Georg Thieme, Leipzig
10. Heinz ER, Yeates A, Burger P et al (1984) Opacification of epidural venous plexus and dura evaluation of cervical spine roots: CT technique. AJNR 5:621–624
11. LaMasters DL, deGroot J (1983) Normal craniocervical junction. In: Newton TH, Potts DG (eds) Computed tomography of the spine and spinal cord. Clavadel Press, St Anselmo, pp 31–52
12. Daniels DL, Williams AL, Haughton VM (1983) Computed tomography of the articulations and ligaments at the occipito-atlanto axial region. Radiology 146:709–716
13. Latchaw RE (1991) MR and CT imaging of the head, neck and spine, 2nd edn. Mosby—year book 1991, CT anatomy of the spine
14. Thijssen A, Keyser MW (1979) Morphology of the cervical spinal cord on computed myelography. Neuroradiology 18:51–62
15. Gillams AR, Soto JA, Carter AP (1997) Fast spin echo vs conventional spin echo in cervical spine imaging. Eur Radiol 7:1211–1214
16. Tsuruda JS, Norman D, Dillon W et al (1989) Three-dimensional gradient-recalled MR imaging as a screening tool for the diagnosis of cervical radiculopathy. AJNR Am J Neuroradiol 10:1263–1271
17. White ML (2000) Cervical spine. MR imaging, techniques and anatomy. MRI Clin North Am 8:453–469
18. Pfirrmann CW, Binkert CA, Zanetti M, Boos N, Hodler J (2001) MR morphology of alar ligaments and occipitoatlantoaxial joints: study in 50 asymptomatic subjects. Radiology 218(1):133–137

Part II

Fractures of the Axis

Demetrios S. Korres

Fractures of the axis are considered to be the commonest injuries of the cervical spine; its position in the upper cervical spine and its anatomy are responsible for that. Data from our department show that the incidence of these fractures is approximately 26.8 % of all cervical spine injuries; men is more often affected, while the average age is noted to be around 45 years.

The cause of these injuries varies. The road traffic accident is by far the commonest cause as more than 61 % of the patients are reported to be involved to this. The second most common cause (34 %) is a fall, either from a high or from body level. Less reported causes (5 %) are related to athletic activities such as diving, boxing, or accidents from weights fallen on the head of a person.

The vast variety of the fractures the axis is subjected is due to its particular anatomy and biomechanical characteristics. The direction of the applied forces as well as the position of the cervical spine and the head has an important role in the creation of the variety of the different types of axis fractures.

The fractures according to the anatomical area involved are divided into five types:

1. Fractures of the odontoid process (49.8 %)
2. Fractures of the vertebral arch, including the spinous and transverse process (36.9 %)
3. Factures of the vertebral body (10.6 %)
4. Isolated fractures of the lateral mass (1.5 %) and
5. A combination of the above fractures (5.1 %).

Hyperextension of the cervical spine is responsible for about 47 % of fractures, hyperflexion accounts for about 26 % and lateral flexion for about 25 %. Less commonly, rotational and compressive forces may, also, be involved. Our experience makes us to note the importance of the knowledge of the direction of the applied force in the spine in order to explain the lesion and proceed to the appropriate movements to treat it. Also, the position of the head at the time of the injury is crucial in the creation of a certain lesion. It is important to consider the possibility of application of more than one force applied to the axis vertebra, a fact that is responsible for the multiple lesions this vertebra may sustained. In the clinical setting, it is very difficult to determine the direction of the applied force, which is usually a combination of subsequently occurring moments responsible for the variety of injuries. It is also worth noting that the axis vertebra is participating in a percentage of about 37 % in double level fractures of the cervical spine or concomitant injuries.

The patient presents with deep pain in the occipital and sub-occipital region, accompanied by cervical stiffness. Pain is exacerbated by pressure on the spinous process of the axis.

D. S. Korres (✉)
University of Athens, 3rd Orthopaedic Department,
KAT Hospital, 10, Heyden Street, 10434, Athens,
Attika, Greece
e-mail: demiskorres@gmail.com

D. S. Korres (ed.), *The Axis Vertebra*,
DOI: 10.1007/978-88-470-5232-1_5, © Springer-Verlag Italia 2013

Fig. 5.1 Open mouth view. Scarcely seen a fracture at the base of the odontoid process (type C1 fracture)

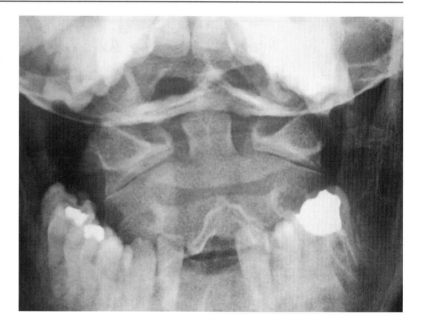

Commonly, a sensory deficit in the form of occipital neuralgia is noted due to pressure on the dorsal branch of the C2 root. Also, rarely, symptoms due to vertebral artery damage or to pressure on the pyramidal tract are seen as well as Wallenberg syndrome or crossed Bell's palsy.

Neurological symptoms due to involvement of the spinal cord are not so common and this because the injury is either lethal due to the involvement of C1, C2 and/or C3 spinal cord segments located posterior to the odontoid process and the body of the axis, or presented with a milder neurological involvement in the form of a spinal cord compression syndrome (i.e. Brown–Sequard) or root compression.

A thorough clinical examination reveals the variety of injuries which accompany these fractures. Head injuries as well as fractures in the axial skeleton are seen in more than 50 % of the cases and may give some information on the direction of the applied force(s).

The diagnosis is based on a thoroughly radiological examination which is described in a previous section. To note, here, the difficulties to clearly imaging of the area of the upper spine and the importance of the knowledge of the normal anatomy and its variants as well as the suspicion of doctors towards underling injury(ies). Special views like the "open mouth" are required for a correct diagnosis (Fig. 5.1)

The main problem of axis fractures is the possibility of instability and the potential threat of life of the injured person. These factors are considered in order to proceed to the appropriate treatment. Nor less important is the fact, that fractures of the axis, may be combined with other injuries, bony or ligamentous, warrant independent consideration. Both, conservative and operative management may be applied to an injured axis vertebra with both options having a place for it.

Although the position of the axis in the upper cervical spine, behind the pharynx is not the best one for direct access, the need for stabilization of certain pattern of fracture led to the development of specific techniques and approaches either anterior, laterally, posterior or combined, so it is possible to reconstruct the fractured axis and to stabilize the spine until solid fusion is achieved.

Apart from the surgical treatment, many authors advocated the conservative management of certain pattern of injuries by using different orthotic constructs.

In both instances, an important role plays the appropriate physiotherapy which will determine the final functional outcome.

Further Reading

Barneschi G (2008) Fratture dell'epistrofeo. In: Traumatologia vertebrale. Verduci Editore, Roma, pp 127–162

Benzel EC, Hart BL, Ball PA et al (1994) Fractures of the C2 vertebral body. J Neurosurg 81:206–212

Fractures of the Odontoid Process

6

Demetrios S. Korres

The incidence of these fractures is around 14 % among the cervical spine fractures and may occur at any age, with a higher risk for patients older than 65 years old, but to note that in this age group, the fracture of the odontoid is more likely to be missed at the initial examination. Progress in diagnostic radiology helped in increasing the number of reported cases. Lambotte, in 1894, was the first to report this type of injury, and at the beginning, only complicated injuries were reported. In the early period, these fractures were managed conservatively, and later in 1910, posterior fixation using a wire was introduced by Mixter and Osgood [1].

The cause of injury is mainly a road traffic accident or a fall, but, other causes are implicated to these injuries. However, the exact prevalence is not known as a certain number of patients sustained such an injury do not survive and are transported dead to the hospital.

The clinical picture of this injury varies from a mild to a severe one (quadriplegia or even death) [2, 3]. The patient is presented in the emergencies holding his head being unable to move it, or is transferred on stretcher complaining of pain in the cervical region. A thorough clinical examination to exclude symptoms corresponding to a neurological damage is needed although there are usually missing. The severity of the neurological disorder corresponds to the degree of displacement and the consequent instability of the odontoid process. Older people have a higher rate of mortality [4].

It is also important to look for an involvement of the vertebral arteries which if damaged could induce symptoms not only at an early stage, but, also, days after the accident.

The understanding of this injury became easier after the experimental studies done the last thirty-five–forty years. Mouradian [5] and Althoff [6] were the first to use cadaveric specimens that included for the first time the whole occipito-atlanto-axial complex. Puttlitz [7] studied in a finite element investigation the probable loading forces and the resulting type of lesion.

The fracture of the odontoid is due often to high-energy trauma with the implication of a combination of forces and the major loading path that cause the lesion is not well established. According to experimental data, the causes of the fractures of the odontoid process are a combination of vertical compression and horizontal shear which acting in a different angle creates different patterns of fracture. In practice, we can assume that the main forces responsible for a fracture of the odontoid process are as follows:

a. Hyper-extension that causes a fracture in the region of the base, in the neck of the dens or in the body of the axis. The odontoid process is hit from the anterior arch of the atlas and a fracture is caused, the direction of which is

D. S. Korres (✉)
University of Athens, 3rd Orthopaedic Department, KAT Hospital, Heyden Street 10, Athens, 10434, Attika, Greece
e-mail: demiskorres@gmail.com

D. S. Korres (ed.), *The Axis Vertebra*,
DOI: 10.1007/978-88-470-5232-1_6, © Springer-Verlag Italia 2013

from anterior-superior toward a posterior-inferior direction.

b. Flexion that leads to a fracture by the sudden and violent blow of the odontoid process by the transverse ligament with a posterior-superior toward anterior-inferior direction of the line fracture.

c. A lateral force, which together with secondary compression and rotational forces, causes a fracture of the neck of the odontoid process as the lateral mass of the atlas hits the dens. The concurrent rotation of the head creates tension in the alar ligaments, which also participate in the creation of this fracture. The rotational force by itself is responsible for the avulsion fractures of the apex of the odontoid process that are created by the sudden contraction of the alar ligaments.

In the majority of cases, the odontoid fractures are due to the application of force in an otherwise normal and healthy cervical spine. Pathological fractures due to an underling pathology the axis vertebra is affected off, are rare, but they do exist [8]. Osteoarthritic alterations at the atlanto-axial joints—which can fix the odontoid process to the anterior arch of the atlas—and at the lower cervical spine are responsible to an increasing risk for fracture at the base of the odontoid process (type B or C) in the elderly persons.

The natural history of dens fracture is not clear, as many factors are involved.

The blood supply of the odontoid process was believed to play an important role in the prognosis of these fractures, but this concept is proven wrong.

An important factor that affects the integrity, the course and the prognosis of these fractures is the degree of their stability. Many authors believe that a fracture that is not accompanied by rupture of the ligaments surrounding the odontoid process or associated fractures of the upper cervical spine and particularly the fractures at the base must be considered as a stable one. In any other case, the fracture is considered to be unstable. Experimental studies carried out under the guidance of Roy-Camille showed that the stability of these fractures depends on the integrity of the posterior longitudinal ligament

and the associated fractures to the axis itself or of the atlas; the latter is responsible for instability in the level between C1 and C2 and the further, in case of fractured pedicles, between C2 and C3 [9].

Knowledge of the pathology of these fractures is crucial in order to assess prognosis and help in the decision we have to make for their management. This led to the development of two basic classification categories according to

a. The position of the fracture.
b. The direction of the line fracture.

In the first category, there are four different classifications described as follows:

1. The Schatzker's classification [10] in which two types are recognized is as follows: (a) the low fracture at the level or below the level of the attachment of the accessory ligaments and (b) the high fracture above the attachment of the accessory ligaments.

2. The Mourgues' classification [11] in which there are two types of fractures. The first is reported to fractures of the base of the odontoid process with a 100 % union prognosis, and the second is reported to fractures at the neck of the odontoid process with a union prognosis of less than 50 %.

3. The Anderson–D'Alonzo classification [12] who proposed the division of the fractures into three types. In the first instance, the authors are reporting to fractures at the top of the odontoid process with a favorable prognosis for union. In the second instance, they are referring to fractures of the neck with a mean rate of pseudarthrosis of about 36 %. The last type the authors are referring is the fractures at the base of the dens. This fracture has a 90 % mean rate of union.

4. The Althoff's classification [6] who proposed four types of dens fractures. The first type with the lesion situated above the neck and having a rate of pseudarthrosis around 64 %. The second type concerns fractures through the neck with a rate of pseudarthrosis of about 55 %. The third type is the one where one of the lateral masses is involved; this lesion has a mean rate of union around 50 % and the fourth type in which the fracture is

situated at the body of the axis vertebra with a high rate of union as 93 %.

The second category, in which the direction of the line is considered, includes the classification of Roy-Camille [1] with four types of fractures as follows:

(a) *Anterior oblique* fractures with posterior-superior toward anterior-inferior direction of the fracture line originating at the level of the neck and directed through the body to the anterior surface of the axis vertebra. This fracture is the result of an impact of the strong transverse ligament on the odontoid process at the time of the applied flexion momentum and represents the commonest type.

(b) *Posterior oblique* fractures with anterior-superior toward posterior-inferior direction of the fracture's line. These fractures are caused by an applied extension momentum, when the anterior rim of the foramen magnum strikes the apex of the odontoid process, and have the tendency to displace posterior.

(c) *Horizontal* fractures with the line of fracture through the neck only; these fractures are the result of the application of a lateral force and are the most unstable.

(d) In some cases, the fracture's line extends to the axis body and becomes transarticular representing the "*English Polishmen's helmet*" [13]. This classification was considered to be the most realistic approach to the determination of, not only the mechanism of creation of the fracture, but also, its stability and prognosis.

The diagnosis of the fractures of the odontoid process relies on the thorough radiological examination, which allows, also, a correct classification.

This is not easy in children and in old people. In children and in young patients, this fracture is rare; we can speak of a separation of the cartilaginous plate with anterior displacement of the odontoid process.

Following the fusion, which will take place at the age of 4–7 years, the picture is completely changed. In adults using conventional radiology, the transoral X-ray may give the most reliable information, while the profile view reveals any

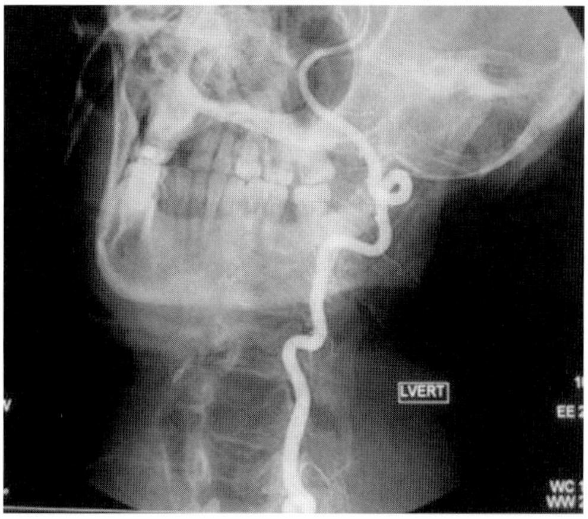

Fig. 6.1 Angiography shows the *left* vertebral artery

anterior or posterior translation or specific findings.

In the case of an undisplaced fracture, the appearance of a pre-vertebral shadow raises the suspicion of an injury.

The vertebral artery if injured may contribute to changes in the clinical picture, so, it is a very important step to be taken for its investigation in order to see any abnormality which would be create problems during manipulations, tractions or even during the operative procedure (Fig. 6.1).

The evolution in the diagnostic methods revealed the existence of other types of fractures, like the vertical one [14–17], and the complex fractures [18, 19]. The vertical fracture is characterized by the division of the odontoid process into two parts with the line fracture extending from the apex to the base while the complex fractures are characterized by a diversity of fractures lines creating the compound or double-level fractures.

Conventional radiological evaluation along with conventional tomography, computerized tomography and 3D scan are considered the best way to identify a fractured odontoid process (Figs. 6.2, 6.3, 6.4, 6.5).

The fractures of the odontoid process represent the mechanical failure of this particular anatomical element following the application of forces [3]. The direction of these forces, the internal architecture, the mechanical strength of the bone trabeculae, the proportion of the

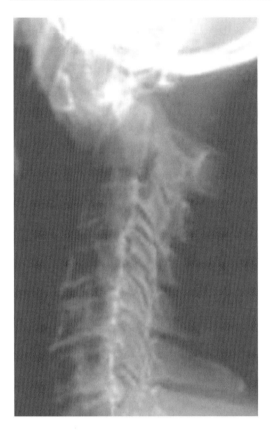

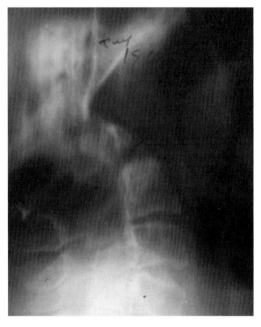

Fig. 6.3 Lateral tomography shows a type B fracture displaced posteriorly

Fig. 6.2 Conventional lateral view

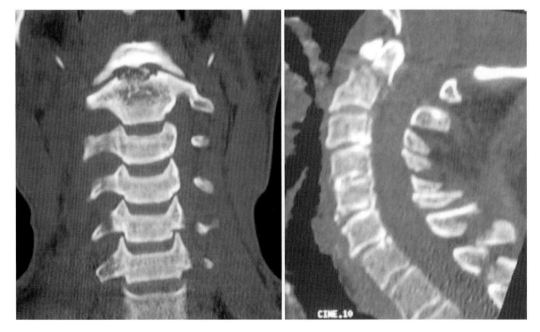

Fig. 6.4 Reconstruction images of a type C1 fracture of the odontoid process with concomitant fractures at C6–C7

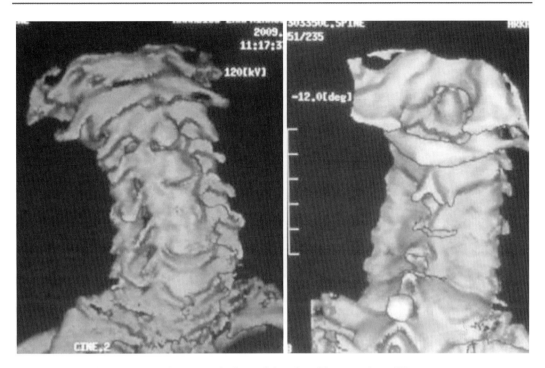

Fig. 6.5 3D scan images show a fracture at the base of the odontoid process (type C1)

cortical and cancellous bone, the magnitude of the odontoid process displacement, the vascular supply of the odontoid process and the age of the patients are the most important factors in the creation of specific fracture types and the prognosis of these injuries.

In line, but not, well documented, in the literature, radiographic and histomorpho-metric studies outlined the structural difference between the odontoid process and the body of the axis. Data from these studies could distinguish the fractures at the base of the odontoid process and the underlying body of the axis.

This was also shown in a recent study using peripheral quantitative computed tomography (pQCT) in cadaveric specimens of the axis [20]. Moreover, this study showed the difference of the internal architecture of the axis between young and older patients; in subjects more than 40 years old, a large void of thin trabecular bone has been identified extending from anterior-inferior to superior-posterior to the base of the odontoid process indicating a mechanically weak region that may predispose to specific fracture patterns [20] (Fig. 6.6).

The Anderson–D'Alonzo classification offers a simple and topographic approach to odontoid process fractures. However, it does not contribute to the thorough understanding of the mechanism of the fracture, nor it incorporates any bio-mechanical characteristics or specific characteristics of the internal architecture of the odontoid process and has limitations [21, 22].

In addition, the many attempts made for its improvement [23, 24] or replacement [3, 8, 10, 25], the existence of alternative classifications based on the direction of the fracture's line [26], the heterogeneity of the reported pseudarthrosis rates at type II fractures and the presence of various unclassified fracture types such as some vertical or oblique fractures [14–16] may suggest the inadequacy of the aforementioned classification schemes.

The classification proposed by Anderson and D'Alonzo is misleading and contributes to confusion regarding fracture location [21]. The Anderson and D'Alonzo type III fracture is not a fracture of the odontoid process, but rather a horizontal rostral fracture through the upper aspect of the body of the axis [21, 22]. Further

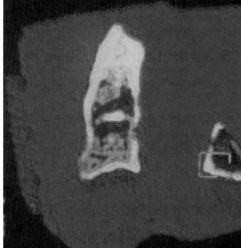

Fig. 6.6 pQCT analysis of the axis vertebra. Note the difference in bone thickness and the void at the posterior part of the base of the odontoid process

adding of subtypes, such as type IIA [23], type IIB [24], type IIC, type II 1–5 [27] and type IIIA [28], perpetuates the confusion. At the same time, Koller stressed the point of a lack of comprehensive classification for fractures of the body and the odontoid process [29].

In the literature, there are fractures not corresponding to the already existing classifications and there is a confusion to be present, so, it is clear that a more appropriate one would be obligatory.

The proposed herein classification is based on the structural, anatomical and bio-mechanical properties of the odontoid process [20, 22].

The anatomical classification we propose accepts four types of fractures and recognizes a zone where practically no fractures are noted (the neutral zone), which is found at the level of transverse ligament, an area of phylogenetically strong bone (Fig. 6.7).

Type A fractures are rare [30, 31]. It is an avulsion fracture at the points of insertion of the alar or apical ligaments with an incidence of 2.3 % in our series; Its stability is questionable, but they responded favorable to a conservative treatment (Fig. 6.8).

Type B fractures represent the most common fractures (38–42 %) of the dens fracture in the literature, and particularly in the elderly population [27] although in our series were second in incidence with 44.1 % (Fig. 6.9). These are the results of lateral force which initiates a rotational movement. In the presence of osteoarthritic changes, this leads easier to a type B or C fracture seeing most frequently in older persons. These fractures represent an unstable lesions with a tendency to pseudarthrosis, so, they need a careful evaluation and appropriate treatment, conservative or surgical, particularly in the old patients [32].

Type C fractures were found to represent 46.6 % [10, 11]; they have a more favorable outcome than type B, responding to a less aggressive management (Figs. 6.10, 6.11).

Finally, *type D* fractures are not so uncommon (7 % in our series) (Fig. 6.12). The axial loading while, the neck is in extension, as well as, a combination of applied forces, which act either simultaneously or not, are probably responsible for this injury. Although it is an unstable lesion, it seems to respond better to a non-surgical treatment.

To note that is easy to recognize a type B from a type C fracture in the lateral view. In type B fracture, the Harris ring is intact as the fracture's line is above this ring. In type C, the fracture line is involving the upper part of the Harris ring (Fig. 6.13, 6.14).

This classification is considered more realistic since it is simple, it includes the whole spectrum of fractures, it refers only to one anatomical structure (the odontoid process), it correlates to the bio-mechanical characteristics of the axis, it indicates the prognosis of the different fracture types and it suggests the adequate evaluation and management of the fractures [22]. Fractures not involving the odontoid process, like the type III in the Anderson–D'Alonzo classification, could not be called odontoid fractures as they are, anatomically speaking, fractures of the axis' body.

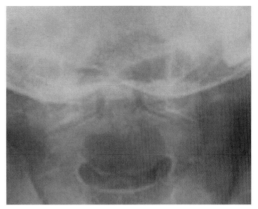

Fig. 6.7 Schematic indication of the level involved at the different fracture patterns. Type A: at the top of the odontoid process. Type B: fractures that occur in the neck of the odontoid process in an area situated below the transverse ligament to a line between the two inner corners of the upper articular processes of the axis. Type C: fractures that occur in the area of the base of the odontoid process between the type B and the anatomical base of the odontoid process are described as type C1. Several fractures extending from the dens itself to the body or at the margins of the lateral masses are classified as type C2 (derooting fractures). Type D: complex fracture (split fractures, comminuted or the double ones) of the odontoid process

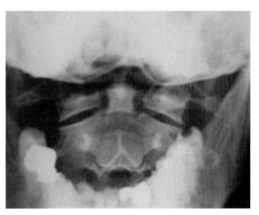

Fig. 6.9 Type B fracture

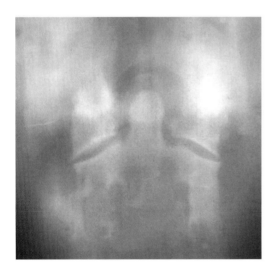

Fig. 6.8 Type A fracture

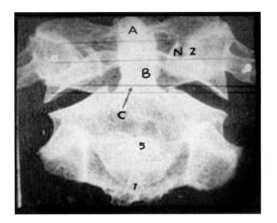

Fig. 6.10 Type C1 fracture

is the presence of the remnants of the subdental synchondrosis. A long debate is still going up [34], but even accepting that the odontoid process is extending down the body of the axis, the lateral articular surfaces are not part of it [35] and the concept of the anatomical reference for an odontoid fracture is stronger [36].

Fractures of the odontoid process should be divided into (a) stable and (b) unstable [1]. This is necessary in order to proceed with the correct therapeutic plan. Stable injuries are managed conservatively, while unstable injuries are treated surgically. Fracture's instability depends mostly on the presence of associated lesions, the type of fracture and the initial displacement, particularly if there is vertical displacement.

Of course, there are many authors who support the concept of Gebauer that the odontoid process is extended down to the body [33]; their argument

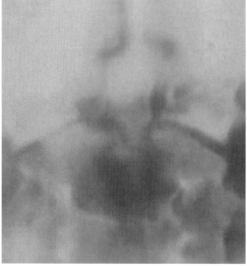

Fig. 6.11 Type C2 fracture

Type A fractures are treated conservatively by using external mobilization, like a rigid cervical collar or a halo vest; rarely an operation should be required.

In type B fractures, although there are unstable, a controversy is still on-going among different authors regarding the surgical approach and management of this lesion [37]. To us an initially conservative treatment should be applied unless a score of more than 10 points is found [38].

In type C, either conservative or operative management is applied in relation to the instability these injuries shown.

In type D, the appropriated conservative management is offering excellent results [16, 19].

Several treatment modalities are proposed in the presence of this injury [39–44], but, before take any decision, it is wise, particularly in the elderly patients, to look for any clinical co morbidities that may affect the management and to rule out any concomitant or double-level fracture of the cervical spine [45, 46].

Conservative treatment is suggested by the use of traction with the application of a Crutchfield skull tongs, in order to reduce and stabilize the fracture or with the use of external immobilization as custom-made orthosis, halo vest or cervical collar.

In case of application of traction, the weight applied should not exceed 2–3 kg, so, as not to distract the fractured fragments. Special care must be given not only to the application of traction, but, also, in its direction. Attention must be paid when traction in flexion is applied, because of the potential danger of a vertebral artery lesion or of a neurological injury which may induce respiratory compromise or other neurological symptoms.

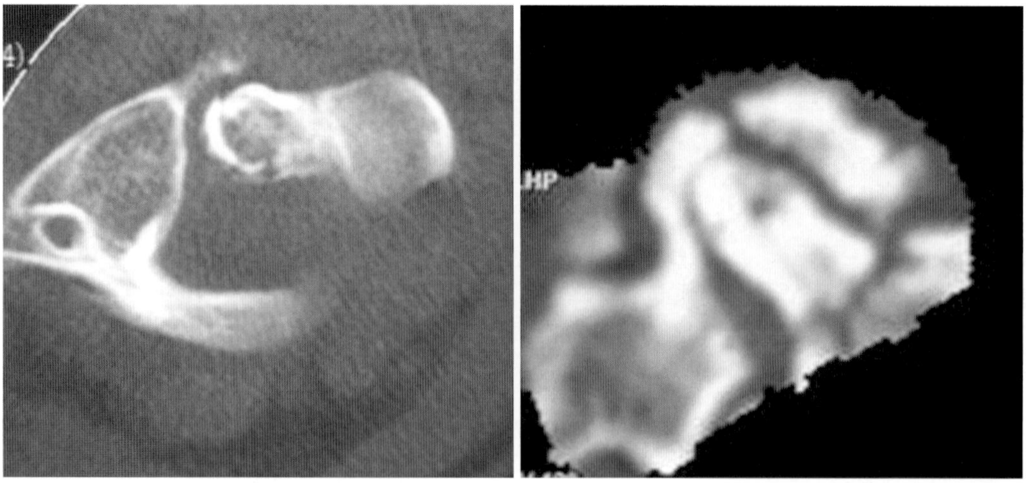

Fig. 6.12 Type D fracture: a split fracture (*left*) and a double fracture (*right*) of the odontoid process (at the base and at the top of the odontoid process)

Fig. 6.13 Type B fracture. **a** Lateral view. Note the fracture's line just above the Harris ring. **b** A–P view of the same patient

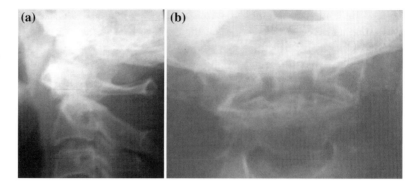

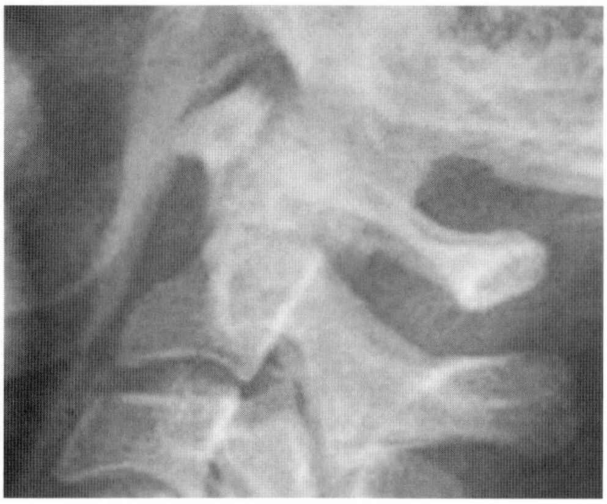

Fig. 6.14 Type C1 fracture. Note the fracture's line crossing the upper part of the Harris' ring

Stabilization must be kept for at least 4–6 weeks during which radiographic control of the position of the fracture is necessary, as well as careful examination for avoidance of complications related to the traction and prolonged bed rest. After this period, the patient may be mobilized using a four-point support brace for a period of four to six more weeks. At the end of 10–12 weeks, dynamic X-ray views in flexion and extension are taken in order to detect any sign of instability. If instability is proven, then, surgical treatment must be considered. If no instability is detected and the fusion is complete, the patient must use a soft collar for a short period of time.

The use of a halo vest is not always recommended as the rate of complications reported is as high as 26 % [47–49] with older persons suffering more from discomfort. Even more, the traction obtained at the beginning is slowly turned into compression, in the mobilized patient, resulting in mal-union, if the reduction of the fracture should be lost due to sliding.

The fusion rate in the conservatively treated patients is reported to be from 35 % as high as 85 % [50], but this is related to the age and other parameters, like the time the treatment was applied, the type of the fracture and the initial displacement; the latter is being correlated with the direction (anterior or posterior) is displaced off.

Also, often, the traction applied leads to distraction at the fracture site; this leads to development of late instability and pseudarthrosis.

Vieweg and Schultheib [51], in contrast to Wolter and Reimann [52], advocate the use of halo vest in type II fractures, as the percentage of healing is as high as 85 %, particularly in the undisplaced ones; they conclude, also, that in type III, the halo vest is the treatment of choice as the rate of healing is about 97 %.

The fractures of the odontoid process are prone to complications either at the trauma scene or later in the hospital.

Two of the complications appearing in a late period are of importance and have to be well clarified: pseudarthrosis and mal-union.

Of importance is the pseudarthrosis, these fractures may develop and the potential danger for late myelopathy [35], or for direct injury of the spinal cord.

According to the literature, the percentage of pseudarthrosis related to the applied treatment is between 4 and 100 % for all types of fractures and consequently complicating their treatment. The predisposing factors which have been accused for pseudarthrosis include age, mechanism of injury, displacement, the blood supply of the odontoid process, the direction of fracture's line and type of fracture. Also, the application of excessive traction, the stability of immobilization, the timing of immobilization, as well as the coexistence of other fracture, either in the atlas or even in the axis itself, play a role [45]. The internal architecture of the axis seems to play an important role in the development of pseudarthrosis [17]. Finally, the possibility of interference of the transverse ligament between the fragments may, also, cause difficulties in the reduction in the fracture, resulting in the development of pseudarthrosis. Some authors may disagree as to the importance of some of the above factors. To our experience, all the above-mentioned factors play a certain role and contribute to the development of pseudarthrosis resulting in instability at the fracture site.

Age has an important role in pseudarthrosis since it has been proved that non-union or pseudarthrosis is found at a higher incidence in patients over the age of 50 years. Fracture displacement according to Blokey and Purser [53] should not be correlated to pseudarthrosis. However, other authors did not accept this opinion. Appuzo et al. [54] described that a shown displacement of more than 4 mm is of significance. However, it is extremely difficult to be aware of the original displacement that was present at the time of the accident.

The traction applied, as well as its direction, play a significant role according to Ryan and Taylor [29]. This is due to the possibility of creating a greater wedging at the fracture level than the one desired, and to lead to a deformed odontoid process.

The type of fracture is also implicated in the development of pseudarthrosis since in fractures involving the neck of the dens as well as the direction of the fracture's line this was in a rate of 32 % and as high as 90 % [55, 56]. In our experience, the types A, C and D are prone to unite, while type B fracture has a high rate of pseudarthrosis, particularly the one that shown a posterior displacement of more than 5 mm or an angulation of more than 10 degrees.

Table 6.1 Factors contributing to pseutharthrosis and their grades

Type of fracture	A	1
	B	6
	C	2
	D	1
Displacement	0 mm	1
	1–6 mm	2
	>7 mm	3
Traction	>4 Kr	1
	<4 Kr	2
Stability	Yes	0
	No	2
Age	<50	1
	>50	2
Associated lesions at the upper cervical spine		2

There is no doubt that the presence of coexisting injuries, as well as a delay in the diagnosis or if the immobilization is not the proper one, then this will increase the instability of the fracture.

The knowledge of these parameters as factors influencing the development of a pseudarthrosis obliged us to proceed in their grading, according to the role each one plays. In this manner, the evaluation of a fracture is more easier, as we will predict the risk for pseudarthrosis [38]. It has been estimated that if the sum of the graded factors is greater than 10 points, then the fracture must be characterized as being at risk of pseudarthrosis and surgical treatment must be considered (Table 6.1).

Pseudarthrosis in the elderly is not always a major problem as it was prevented [22, 50] that this is not accompanied always by a clinically significant instability due to the development of fibrous tissue at the fracture site (Fig. 6.15). However, operation has to be considered if instability persists or if signs of myelopathy are elicited.

Operative treatment of dens non-unions is not without risk, taking into consideration the age of the patients the high comorbidity those patients have and, also, knowing that the success rate is low.

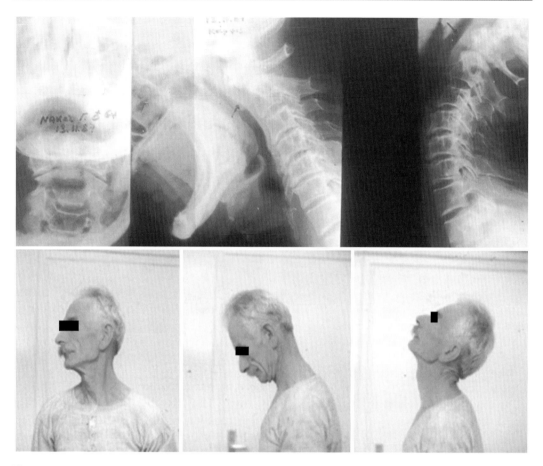

Fig. 6.15 Pseudarthrosis of a type B fracture. 27 years later, there is mobility at the fracture's site, and the fracture's line is still visible, there is no instability in flexion—extension dynamic views, and the patient has a full range of neck motion without complains

The second most frequent and severe complication of the fractures of the odontoid process concerns their mal-union [57, 58] (Fig. 6.16). Special care so must be given to this complication as may result in spinal canal stenosis which may induce, in long term, cervical myelopathy.

The greater the displacement and wedging of the fracture, the less the width of the spinal canal. This results in chronic compression or friction of the dura matter and the spinal cord on the upper posterior corner of the body of the axis and hence cervical myelopathy [59]. The treatment of this complication is difficult. It requires anterior or posterior decompression combined with posterior fusion extending from the occipital bone to C1, C2 or C3 and even lower.

A number of minor complications may accompany a fractured odontoid. Stiffness, decreased range of movements, discomfort or even mild pain are easily managed with physiotherapy or other conservative methods. younger patients response better, and an uneventful outcome is usually achieved.

Failure to treat conservatively a fractured odontoid is an indication for surgical intervention [60, 61].

Instability must be treated operatively as soon as possible. The operative approach is suggested by many authors [41, 42, 62–64]. There are several methods that allow the safe management of the unstable fractures. This is done by closed or open reduction, the use of osseous graft and stabilization by means of a wire or nylon or use

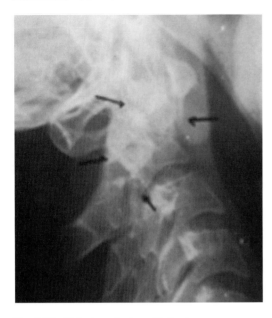

Fig. 6.16 Malunion of a type C1 fracture

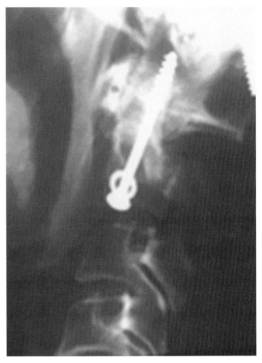

Fig. 6.18 Anterior osteosynthesis

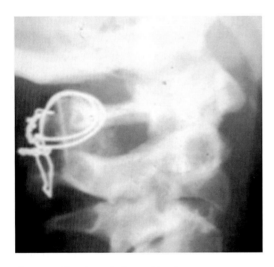

Fig. 6.17 Brooks technique with wires

of implant(s). Auto-graft is the most suitable material to be used for achievement of a stable fusion. The approach used is anterior, lateral, posterior or combined.

Posterior stabilization includes as follows:

Posterior C1–C2 wiring technique with Gallie's or Brooks' techniques or other methods [1, 40, 41, 64–67] (Fig. 6.17). The posterior C1–C2 screw fixation is reported to be effective in case of unstable odontoid fractures and for

other pathologies, like atlanto-axial dislocation or Jefferson fractures. Using these techniques, we can stabilize the C1–C2 level, but the disadvantage of a potential injury to the vertebral arteries and the limitation of the range of movements of the neck are reality.

Anterior stabilization includes:

a. Application of a plate between the anterior arch of the atlas and the body of the axis or the vertebral body of C3 [68, 69]

b. Internal fixation with screw(s) [43, 70, 71] (Fig. 6.18). This technique is gaining popularity, but indications have to be set very carefully as osteoporosis, fracture of the anterior wall of the body of C2, posterior displacement, comminuted or type D fractures or even a narrow diameter of the spinal canal are among the contraindications. The osteosynthesis of the odontoid process permits a nearly normal function of the C1–C2 level.

Lateral stabilization includes as follows:

Fusion using the Dutoit technique [72, 73]. The lateral approach is used for a C1–C2 arthrodesis in case of traumatic instability,

Table 6.2 Indications for treatment of an odontoid fracture

Type A	Conservative
Type B	Conservative/surgical
Type C1	Conservative/surgical
Type C2	Conservative
Type D	Conservative

tumors or infections and for cases in which other, previously used approach, or a counter-indication is present.

The surgical results seem to be better than those achieved with a non-operative management as the reported fusion rate is high between 80 and 100 %. However, there is not unanimous acceptance of an appropriate treatment of patients with these fractures, particularly in the elderly population. Table 6.2 summarizes the indications for the appropriated management of an odontoid fracture.

The physiotherapist or physical training instructor, has an important role to play in the final outcome those patients should have. The rehabilitation protocol generally includes three phases. In the first phase (in-hospital), we use the ergonomy position on the bed. In the second phase, following removal of the sutures, gentle range of motion exercises of the cervical spine is started, followed by progressive increase in the range of motion and strengthening exercises of the neck muscles as tolerated. Finally, in the third phase (2–3 months post-injury), increased activities are allowed including aerobics, swimming pool and exercises of the upper thoracic muscles. Patients' compliance remains the key for a final acceptable outcome.

References

1. Roy-Camille R, Lepresie PH, Mazel Chr (1986) Les fractures de l'odontoide In : Roy-Camille (ed) Rachis cervical supérieure Masson Cie Paris, pp 99–118
2. Barnechi G (2008) Fratture dell'epistrofeo. In: Barneschi G (ed) Traumatologia vertebrale. Verduci editore, Roma, pp 127–162
3. Crockard HA, Heilman AE, Stevens JM (1993) Progressive myelopathy secondary to odontoid fractures, clinical, radiological and surgical features. J Neurosurgery 78:579–586
4. Malik SA, Murphy M, Connolly P et al (2008) Evaluation of morbidity, mortality and outcome following cervical spine injuries in elderly patients. Eur Spine J 17:585–591
5. Mouradian WH, Fiett VG, Cochran GVB, Fielding JW, Young J (1978) Fractures of the odontoid: a laboratory and clinical study of mechanisms. Orthop Clin N Am 9:985–1001
6. Althoff B, Bardholm H (1979) Fractures of the odontoid process. An experimental and clinical study. Acta Orthop Scand Suppl 177:1–91
7. Puttlitz CM, Goel VK, Clark CR, Traynelis VC (2000) Pathomechanisms of failures of the odontoid. Spine 25:2868–2876
8. Klemola R, Karttunen A, Laine M et al (2000) Nontraumatic dens fracture in a patient with lymphangiomatosis: radiographic, CT, and MRI findings. Emerg Radiol 8:119–122
9. Roy-Camille R, Lafosse L, Bouchet Th, Judet Th (1986) Les associations traumatiques du rachis cervical superieur. In: Roy-Camille R (ed) Rachis cervical superieure. Parispp, Masson, pp 137–141
10. Schatzker J, Rorabeck CH, Waddell JP (1971) Fractures of the dens (odontoid process): an analysis of thirty-seven cases. J Bone Joint Surg Br 53:392–405
11. De Mourgues G, Fischer LP, Bejui J, Carret JP, Gonon GP, Subasi H (1981) Fracture of the odontoid process [in French]. Rev Chir Orthop Reparatrice Appar Mot 67:783–790
12. Anderson LD, D'Alonzo RT (1974) Fractures of the odontoid process of the axis. J Bone Jt Surg Am 56:1663–1674
13. Roy-Camille R, de la Caffiniere J-Y, Saillant G (ed) (1973) Traumatismes du rachis cervical supérieur C1–C2. Masson, Paris
14. Bergenheim T, Forssell A (1991) Vertical odontoid fracture-case report. J Neurosurg 74:665–667
15. Johnson JE, Yang PJ (1986) Vertical fracture of the odontoid: CT diagnosis. Neurosurg 23:31–35
16. Castillo M, Mukherji SK (1996) Vertical fracture of the dens. AJNR Am J Radiol 17:1627–1630
17. Kokkino AJ, Lazio BE, Perin NI (1996) Vertical fracture of the odontoid process: case report. Neurosurgery 38:200–203
18. Korres DS, Babis G, Evangelopoulos D-S et al (2008) Combined double fractures of the odontoid process and fracture of the atlas: a case report. Eur J Orthop Surg Traumatol 14:34–36
19. Korres DS, Mavrogenis AF, Gratsias P et al (2010) Type D fractures of the odontoid process. Eur J Orhop Surg Traumatol 20:597–601
20. Korres DS, Karachalios T, Roidis N et al (2004) Structural properties of the axis vertebra. Clin Orthop Rel Res 418:134–140

21. Benzel EC, Hart BL, Ball PA, Baldwin NG, Orrison WW, Espinosa M (1994) Fractures of the C2 vertebral body. J Neurosurgery 81:206–212

22. Korres DS, Mavrogenis AF, Gratcias P, Lyritis GP, Papagelopoulos PJ (2008) It is time to reconsider the classification of dens fractures. Eur J Orthop Surg Traumatol 18:189–195

23. Hadley MN, Brown CM, Liu SS, Sonntag VKH (1988) New subtype of acute odontoid fractures (type IIA). Neurosurgery 22:67–71

24. Gauer JN, Shaft B, Hilibrand AS et al (2005) Proposal of a modified, treatment-oriented classification of odontoid fractures. Spine J 5:123–129

25. Roy-Camille R, Saillant G, Judet TH, Botton G, Michel G (1980) Elements de prognostic des fractures de l' odontoide. Rev Chir Orthop Reparatrice Appar Mot 66:183–186

26. Katoh S, El Masry WS, Inman CG (1994) Oblique odontoid fracture: case report and review of the literature. Paraplegia 32:108–111

27. Reihold M, Bellabarba C, Bransford R, Chapman J et al (2011) Radiographic analysis of type II odontoid fractures in a geriatric patient population: description and pathomechanism of the "Geier"-deformity. Eur Spine J 20:1928–1939. doi:10.1007/s00586-011-1903-6

28. Jea A, Tatsui Cl, Farhat H, Vanni S, Levi AD (2006) Vertically unstable type III odontoid fractures: case report. Neurosurgery 58:E797

29. Koller H, Kammermeier V, Assunca A, Holz U (2007) Spinal Stenosis C1-2 following redo surgery for failed odontoid screw fixation—scrutinizing the odontoid fracture classification. Internet J Spine Surg 3:1–11

30. Scott EW, Haid RW Jr, Peace D (1990) Type I fractures of the odontoid process: implication for atlanto-occipital instability. Case report. J Neurosurg 72:488–492

31. Yanagawa Y, Takemoto M, Takasu A, Sakamoto T et al (2005) Type I odontoid fracture—case report. Neurol Med Chir (Tokyo) 45:92–96

32. Ryan MD, Taylor TK (1993) Odontoid fractures in the elderly. J Spinal Disord 6:397–401

33. Gebauer M, Barvencik F, Beil FT, Lohce C, Pogoda P, Puschel K, Rueger JM, Amling M (2007) Die Subdentale sychondrose. Unfalchirurg 110:97–103

34. Wang XP, Deng ZC, Liang ZI, Tu YM (2008) Response to reply to the letter to the editor concerning "Gebauer et al: subdental synchondrosis and anatomy of the axis in the aging: a histomorphometric study on 30 autopsy cases". Eur Spine J 15:292–298, The basis of the dens axis. Where it is located? Eur Spine J 17:1771–1774, author reply, pp 1775–1776

35. Aug Wankenheim (1989) Imagerie du rachis cervical I. Springer, Wien

36. Gray H (1918) The cervical vertebrae osteology. Gray's Anatomy of the Human body

37. Denaro V, Papalia R, Di Martino A, Denaro L, Maffulli N (2011) The best surgical treatment for type II fractures of the dens is still controversial. Rev Clin Orthop Relat Res 469:742–750

38. Korres DS, Stamos KG, Andreakos AG, Hardouvelis Chr, Kouris A (1989) Fractures of the dens and risk of pseudarthrosis. Arch Orthop Trauma Surg 108:373–376

39. Blondel B, Philippe M, Fuentes S, Dutertre G, Dufour H (2009) Single anterior procedure for stabilization of a three-part fracture of the axis (odontoid dens and hangman fracture). Case report. Spine 34:E255–E257

40. Buchholz RD, Cheung KC (1989) Halo vest versus spinal fusion for cervical injury: evidence from an outcome study. J Neurosurg 70:884–892

41. Jeanneret B, Magerl F (1992) Primary posterior fusion of C1/2 in odontoid fractures: indication, techniques and results of transarticular facet screw fixation. J Spinal Disord 5:464–475

42. Platzer P, Thalhammer G, Ostermann R et al (2007) Anterior screw fixation of odontoid fractures comparing younger and elderly patients. Spine 32:1714–1720

43. Platzer P, Thalhammer G et al (2009) Plate fixation of odontoid fractures without C1–C2 arthrodesis: practice of a novel technique for stabilization of odontoid fractures, including the opportunity to extend the fusion. Neurosurgery 64:726–733

44. Yong YLY, Fu BS, Rachel WL et al (2011) Anterior single screw fixation of odontoid fracture with intraoperative iso-C 3-dimensional imaging. Eur Spine J 20:1899–1907

45. Korres DS et al (1987) Double level fractures of the cervical spine. Int Ortop 11:105–108

46. Hanigan WC, Powell FC, Elwood PW et al (1993) Odontoid fractures in elderly patients. J Neurosurg 78:32–35

47. Glaser JA, Whitehill R, Stamp WG, Jane JA (1986) Complications associated with the halo vest. A review of 265 cases. J Neurosurg 65:762–769

48. Evangelopoulos DS, Kontovazenitis P, Kokkinis K, Efstathopoulos N, Korres DS (2009) Symptomatic intracranial abscess after treating lower cervical spine fracture with halo vest: a case report and review of literature. Case J 2:101

49. Lind B, Nordwall A, Sihlbohm H (1987) Odontoid fractures treated with halo vest. Spine 12:173–177

50. Molinari RW, Khera OA, Gruhn WL, MacAssey RW (2012) Rigid cervical collar treatment for geriatric type II odontoid fractures. Eur Spine J 21:855–862. doi:10.1007/s00586-011-2069-y

51. Vieweg U, Schultheiss A (2001) A review of halo vest treatment of the upper cervical spine injuries. Arch Orthop Truma Surg 121:50–55

52. Wolter D, Reimann B (1989) Possibilities and limits of the therapy of cervical spine injuries with the halo. Unfallchirurgie 15:83–94

53. Blockey NJ, Purser DW (1956) Fractures of the odontoid process of the axis. J Bone Joint Surg 38-B:794–816

54. Apuzzo MLJ, Heiden JS, Weiss MH, Ackerson TT, Harvey JP, Kurze T (1978) Acute fractures of the odontoid process–an analysis of 45 cases. J Neurosurg 48:85–91

55. Clark CR, White AA (1985) Fractures of the dens. J Bone Joint Surg Am 67:1340–1348

56. Roy-Camille R, Saillant G, Lepresie PH, Leonard P (1983) Fractures récentes de l'odontoide. Presse Med 12:2233–2236

57. Heller JG, Levy MJ, Barrow DL (1993) Odontoid fracture malunion with fixed atlantoaxial subluxation. Spine 18:311–314

58. Ho Angela W-H, Ho Y-F (2010) Atlanto-axial deformity secondary to a neglected odontoid fracture: a report of six cases. J Orthop Surg 18:235–240

59. Fairholm D, Lee ST, Lui TN (1996) Fractrured odontoid: the management of delayed neurological symptoms. Neurosurgery 38:38–43

60. Kanaoutas E, Ambrozaitis KV, Spakauskas Kalesinskas RJ (2005) The treatment of odontoid fractures with significant displacement. Medcina (Kaunas) 41:23–29

61. Kuntz C IV, Mirza SK, Jarell AD et al (2000) Type II odontoid fractures in the elderly: early failure of nonsurgical treatment. Neurosurg Focus 8:e7

62. Al Vaccaro, Matigan L, Ehrler DM (2000) Contemporary management of adults cervical odontoid fractures. Orthopedics 23:1109–1113

63. Fountas NK, Kapsalaki EZ, Karampelas I et al (2005) Results of long-term follow-up in patients undergoing anterior screw fixation for type II and rostral type III odontoid fractures. Spine (Phila Pa 1976) 30:661–669

64. Frangen TM, Zilkens C, Muhr G et al (2007) Odontoid fractures in the elderly: dorsal C1/C2 fusion is superior to halo-vest immobilization. J Trauma 63:83–89

65. Brooks AL, Jenkins EB (1978) Atlanto-axial arthrodesis by the wedge compression method. J Bone Joint Surg 60-A:279–284

66. Harms J, Melcher RP (2001) Posterior C1–C2 fusion with polyaxial screw and rod fixation. Spine (Phila Pa 1976) 26:2467–2471

67. Lehman RA, Sasso RC (2007) Current concepts in posterior C1–C2 fixation. Semin Spine Surg 19(4):244–249

68. Streli R (1987) Dens transfixation plate. In: Kehr P, Weidner A (ed) Cervical spine I. Springel, pp 239–243

69. Yin QS, Ai FZ, Zhang K (2004) Design ad preliminary clinical application of trasoralpharygeal atlanto-axial plate. Zhonghua Wai Ke Za Zhi 42:1325–1329

70. Muller EJ, Wick M, Russe OJ, Palta M, Muhr G (2000) Anterior screw fixation for odontoid fractures. Unfallch 103:38–43

71. Jian Wang, Yue Zhou, Zhang ZF, Li CQ, Zheng WJ (2011) Comparison of percutaneous and open anterior screw fixation in the treatment of type II and rostral type III odontoid fractures. Spine 36:1459–1463

72. Du Toit G (1976) Lateral atlanto-axial arthrodesis: a screw fixation technique. S Afr J Surg 14:9–12

73. Feron J-M (1981) Abord chirurgical latérale des massifs articulaires de l'atlas et de l'axis. Technique et indications. Thèse Medecin, Paris

Fractures of the Vertebral Body

Demetrios S. Korres and Nikolaos E. Efstathopoulos

Fractures of the body of the axis represent a separate entity; the body itself is an anatomical area well recognized. Many authors paid particular attention and have already described these lesions [1–10]. Initially, authors referred to as a non-hangman, non-odontoid fracture [11, 12], but we believe that these fractures could be covered under one label that is *fractures of the body of the axis*. This lesion is frequent, accounting for about 11 % in our series.

Many attempts were undertaken to classify the fractures of the body of the axis. Benzel [12] in 1994 recognized three types according to the orientation of the fracture: the coronal, the sagittal, and the horizontal ones. Fijimura in 1996 [4] proposed four types according to the imaging: avulsion fracture, transverse, burst, and sagittal ones. Craig and Hodgson in 1991 [13] as well as Hähnle in 1999 [7] added the shearing type of lesion that is the anterior or lateral part of the axis together with the odontoid process separated from the rest of the body. There is no doubt that as the axis body is subjected to a

diversity of applied forces, the lesion that is to be done is out of any planned model and the variety of lesion is apparent, like the lesion described by us [14]. The following patterns of fractures have been distinguished:

a. tear drop fractures of the axis (or avulsion),
b. transverse fractures of the body,
c. vertical, and
d. miscellaneous.

a. Tear drop fractures involve the anterior inferior corner of the vertebral body (Fig. 7.1). They are characterized by an avulsed fragment, of varying size, from the anterior inferior angle of the body of the axis as a result of hyperextension usually following a road traffic accident. This type of injury is not frequent, representing 3 % of all cervical spine trauma.

Tear drop fractures of the axis are due to hyperextension, leading to compression of the posterior bony elements which then act as a fulcrum. The avulsion fracture of the anterior lower angle of the vertebral body is caused by distension of the anterior longitudinal ligament. The fracture line extends from the anterior part of the vertebral body, backwards and downwards to the inferior end plate of the axis. The injury also leads to rupture of the intervertebral disc at the C2–C3 level from the junction of the disc and the fracture line, which then extends backwards. If the hyperextension force persists, the injury may extend to the posterior ligamentous elements, which may result in a posterior displacement of the body of the axis [15], and injury to the spinal cord; the latter is quite rare.

D. S. Korres (✉)
3rd Orthopaedic Department, KAT Hospital,
University of Athens, Heyden 10, 104 34, Athens,
Attika, Greece
e-mail: demiskorres@gmail.com

N. E. Efstathopoulos
2nd Orthopaedic Department, Konstantopoulion
Hospital, University of Athens, Agias Olgas 3, 142
33, Nea Ionia, Attika, Greece
e-mail: nefstatho@med.uoa.gr

D. S. Korres (ed.), *The Axis Vertebra*,
DOI: 10.1007/978-88-470-5232-1_7, © Springer-Verlag Italia 2013

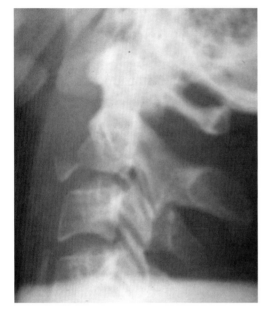

Fig. 7.1 Tear drop fracture of the axis

These lesions are better managed conservatively in a hard collar. The injury is accompanied very often with a second fracture either of the axis itself or of at another level (Fig. 7.2) [3].

The stability of the injury has been questioned [15], but we believe that, in spite of the size of the avulsed fragment or its displacement, this fracture remains a stable lesion with a good prognosis.

The treatment of choice in the case of an isolated "tear drop" fracture is conservative, that is, immobilization, followed by the application of a hard cervical collar, or a halo vest. Operative treatment advocated by some authors [15–17] seems to have no place. The presence of a coexisting lesion may sometimes require a more rigid and prolonged immobilization.

b. Transverse or horizontal fractures (Fig. 7.3). The peculiar anatomy of the axis as well as its internal architecture, together with specific biomechanical responses, leads to different patterns of fractures of the body. Forces like hyperextension alone or combined with flexion are responsible for horizontal fractures of the body which could presented in three ways:

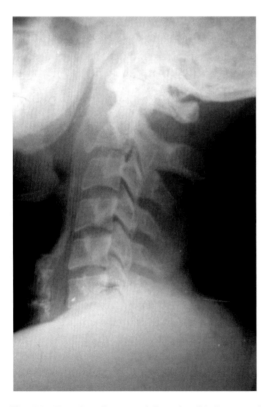

Fig. 7.2 Tear drop fracture of the axis with fracture of the spinous process of C6

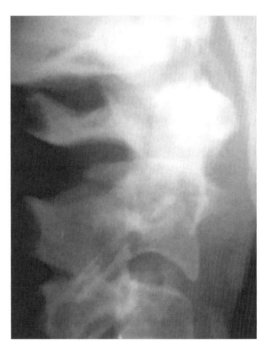

Fig. 7.3 Horizontal fracture (Chance type) of the body of the axis

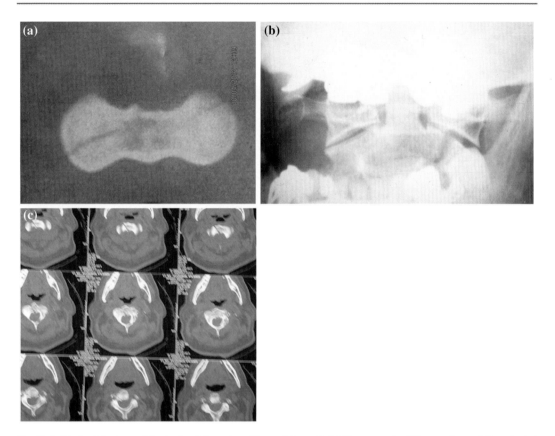

Fig. 7.4 Vertical fracture of the body of the axis. **a** Coronal, **b** sagittal CT scan, and **c** CT scan of a sagially oriented fracture

a. as a fracture starting at the anterior wall of the axis and extending parallel to the lower surface of the body, towards the posterior wall, below the pedicles,

b. as a fracture extending from the anterior wall posteriorly through the body and the posterior arch, representing a Chance type of fracture, and

c. as a fracture extending from the posterior wall anteriorly at the upper aspect of the vertebral body, representing the previously described by Anderson-D' Allonzo as type III fracture of the odontoid process.

All these patterns of fracture, although described in the literature [1, 4, 6, 12, 18], are very uncommon. These fractures although represent a potentially unstable lesion, their prognosis is good, responding well to a non-operative treatment.

c. Vertical fractures . These are fractures created from excessive axial loading. There are two sub-groups:

a. the vertical fracture with a coronal orientation (Fig. 7.4a) and

b. the vertical fracture presenting with a sagittal oriented lesion (Fig. 7.4b).

Benzel in 1994 [12] described the mechanism involved (axial loading); the position of the head will determine the pattern of fractures, as it is the factor which will indicate the area the force will hit the axis vertebra. CT scan reconstruction is a useful tool to understand the type of injury (Fig. 7.4c).

d. Miscellaneous. This group includes a variety of fractures which result after the application of force in certain direction and depending on the position of the axis vertebra in

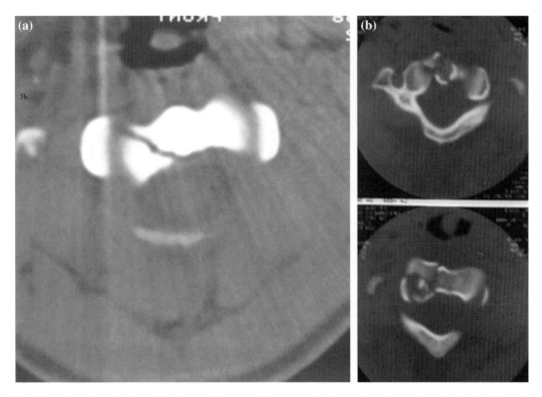

Fig. 7.5 **a** Shear-type fracture of the body of the axis. **b** Compound fracture of the lateral side of the body of the axis

relation to the head and in relation to the rotation the neck had at the time of injury. Therefore, there are fractures described as shear fractures, oblique, far laterally vertical, compound or multiple (Fig. 7.5a, b) [6–8].

A shear-type fracture is due to asymmetrical axial compression [7], while hyperextension with additional lateral flexion or rotation is believed to be the mechanism of an oblique fracture [19]. An axial force combined with lateral bending and rotation can also lead to collapse of the lateral mass [6]. The weak point for explanation of the mechanism of these fractures is the small series published till now that cannot permit to draw valuable conclusions.

Meanwhile, it seems to be an agreement as far as the management of these lesions is concern. Conservative treatment with a halo vest should be attempted initially, and in case of failure of reduction or fracture displacement, atlantoaxial

fusion is recommended. The involvement of the joints in certain of these fractures will lead sooner or later to arthritic alterations.

References

1. Maki NJ (1985) A transverse fracture through the body of the axis—a case report. Spine 10:857–859
2. Bohay D, Gosselin RA, Contreras D (1992) The vertical axis fracture: a report on three cases. J Orthop Trauma 6:416–419
3. Korres DS, Zoubos AB, Kavadias K, Babis GC, Balalis K (1994) The "tear drop" (or avulsed) fracture of the anterior inferior angle of the axis. Eur Spinal J 3:151–154
4. Fujimura Y, Nishi Y, Kobayashi K (1996) Classification and treatment of axis body fractures. J Orthop Trauma 10:536–540
5. Greene KA, Dickman CA, Marciano FF et al (1997) Acute axis fractures: analysis of management and outcome in 340 consecutive cases. Spine 22(16):1843–1852

6. Jakim J, Sweet MBE (1998) Transverse fracture through the body of the axis. J Bone Joint Surg 70-B:728–729
7. Hähnle U, Wisniewski TF, Craig JB (1999) Shear fracture through the body of the axis vertebra. Spine 24:2278–2281
8. American Association of Neurological Surgeons (2002) Isolated fractures of the axis in adults. Neurosurgery 50(Suppl 3):105–147
9. German JW, Hart BL, Benzel EC (2005) Nonoperative management of vertical C2 body fractures. Neurosurgery 56:516–521
10. Watanabe M, Kanno T, Komada W, Miura H, Foxton RM, Tagami J (2011) Clinical features of the extension tear drop fracture of the axis: review of 13 cases. J Neurosurg Spine 14(6):710–714
11. Johnson JE, Yang PJ (1986) Vertical fracture of the odontoid: CT diagnosis. Neurosurgery 23:31–35
12. Benzel EC, Hart BL, Ball PA, Baldwin NG, Orrison WW, Espinosa M (1994) Fractures of the C2 vertebral body. J Neurosurg 81:206–212
13. Craig JB, Hodgson BF (1991) Superior facet fractures of the axis vertebra. Spine 16:875–877
14. Korres DS, Papagelopoulos PJ, Mavrogenis AF, Sapkas GS, Patsinevelos A, Kyriazopoulos P, Evangelopoulos D (2004) Multiple fractures of the axis. Orthopedics 27:1096–1099
15. Mazel CHR, Roy-Camille R (1990) Tear drop fractures of C2-pathogenesis and treatment. Abstracts of 7th annual meeting of the CSRS. Taormina, Italy. Paper No 37, p 81
16. Dhinsa SB, Agarwal A, Prsar RV, Morar Y, Hammer A (2011) Anterior plating for an axis tear drop fracture: a case report. Eur Orthop Traumatol. doi:10.1007/s12570-011-0049-7
17. Vialle R, Schmider L, Levassor N, Rilardon L, Drain O, Guigui P (2004) Extension tear drop–drop fracture of the axis: a surgically treated case. Rev Orthop Reparatrice Appar Mot 90:152–155
18. Korres DS, Papagelopoulos PJ, Mavrogenis A, Benetos J, Kyriazopoulos P, Gavras GM (2005) Chance type fracture of the axis. Spine 30(17):E517–E520
19. Goldschlager T, Leach JCD, Williamson OD, Malham G (2010) Oblique axis body fracture—pitfalls in management. Inj Int J Care 43(4):505–508

Fractures of the Posterior Arch

8

Efstratios Kavroudakis and Demetrios S. Korres

Fractures of the posterior arch of the axis vertebra may include the pedicles (unilateral or bilateral) or the spinous process (Fig. 8.1); the latter are uncommon, do not cause any serious complications and are associated with an uneventful outcome. Of greater importance are the fractures occurring at the anatomic area of the pars interarticularis. In such cases, one has to deal with a traumatic spondylolisthesis, a serious injury frequently seen in the emergency rooms. For this type of injury, instead of hangman's fracture, we prefer to use the term traumatic spondylolisthesis of the axis.

8.1 Traumatic Spondylolisthesis of the Axis

Traumatic spondylolisthesis of the axis is the second most common fracture of the second cervical vertebra (C2) with an incidence of about 37 %. It involves a bilateral fracture of the pars interarticularis with variable displacement and angulation of the C2 over the C3 vertebra.

It was described by Haughton in 1866 [1] who studied the cervical spine of persons executed by hanging. Garber in 1964 [2] was the first to use the term "traumatic spondylolisthesis of the axis". Biomechanically, four types of forces contribute to the development of such fractures, acting either separately or in combination: hyperextension, traction, compression and flexion. Two distinct mechanisms are reported. The first is the result of a combined hyperextension-compression-flexion force, as in the case of a person falling from a height and landing with the face towards the ground or of a victim of a traffic accident hitting the frontal glass of the car with his head. The second mechanism is the result of a hyperextension-traction force as in the originally described hangman's fracture.

The common feature in both fracture mechanisms is the hyperextension and is probably the causative factor of the initial injury (rupture of the anterior longitudinal ligament). The inferior articular process of the axis collides with the superior articular process of C3 resulting in fracture of the pars interarticularis of the axis with or without avulsion fracture of the anterior surface of C2 or C3.

If hyperextension is followed by a flexion force (like in a whiplash injury), the intervertebral disc may be detached, more commonly from the body of C3 and less often from the body of the axis leading to rupture of the posterior longitudinal ligament and consequent

D. S. Korres (✉)
3rd Orthopaedic Department, KAT Hospital,
University of Athens, Heyden 10, 10434, Athens,
Attika, Greece
e-mail: demiskorres@gmail.com

E. Kavroudakis
3rd Orthopaedic Department, KAT Hospital,
University of Athens, Zafeiriou 4, 17122, Nea
Smyrni, Attika, Greece
e-mail: ekavroudakis@hotmail.com

D. S. Korres (ed.), *The Axis Vertebra*,
DOI: 10.1007/978-88-470-5232-1_8, © Springer-Verlag Italia 2013

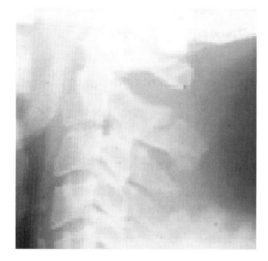

Fig. 8.1 Fracture of the spinous process of the axis

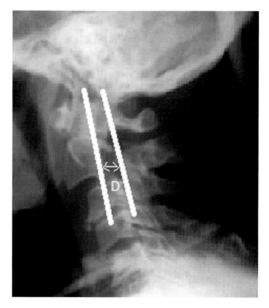

Fig. 8.2 The anterior dislocation (D) of the fracture is calculated by measuring the distance between the two lines that run parallel to the posterior border of the axis and C3 at the level of C2–C3 intervertebral space (Courtesy of Dr Zachariou)

anterior translation of the body of the axis. If the flexion force persists, dislocation of the articular processes also occurs [3].

Three main classifications have been reported for the traumatic spondylolisthesis of the axis: (1) Effendi's classification, (2) Francis' classification, and (3) Levine and Edwards' classification. Effendi's classification [4] of traumatic spondylolisthesis of the axis and its modification by Levine and Edwards [5] is based on the degree of angular deformity and anterior dislocation of the axis with respect to the body of C3 (Figs. 8.2, 8.3). Type I (69 % in our series) refers to bilateral fractures of the pars interarticularis with anterior dislocation of <3 mm and no angulation (Fig. 8.4). It represents a stable injury that does not increase with flexion and that is reduced with extension of the cervical spine. The mechanism of injury is a combination of hyperextension and axial compression. A small avulsion fracture of the anterior rim of C3 or the posterior lower rim of the axis may be present as well. Moreover, other injuries that are due to hyperextension may coexist, such as fracture of the posterior arch of the atlas (C1), Jefferson's fracture, fracture of the lateral mass of C1 and fracture of the odontoid process [6]. Type II (27 %) is characterized by an anterior dislocation of the axis of >3 mm and significant angulation of >11° (Fig. 8.5). There is concomitant rupture of the C2–C3 intervertebral

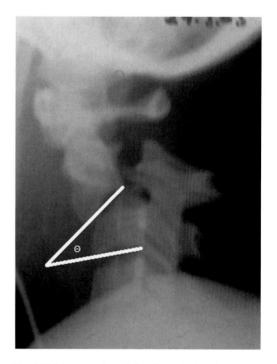

Fig. 8.3 The angular deformity of the fracture is measured by the angle (Θ) that forms between the lines that run parallel to the inferior epiphyseal plates of the axis and C3

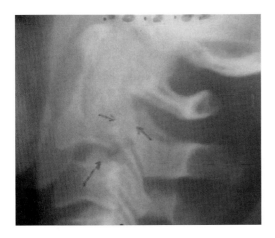

Fig. 8.4 Effendi's type I traumatic spondylolisthesis

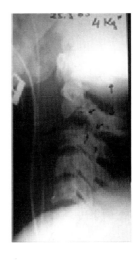

Fig. 8.6 Effendi's type III traumatic spondylolisthesis

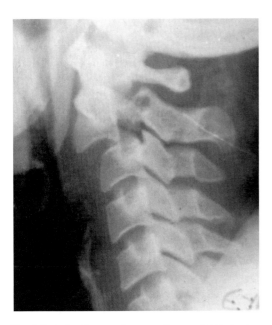

Fig. 8.5 Effendi's type II traumatic spondylolisthesis

disc and the posterior longitudinal ligament. The anterior longitudinal ligament remains intact, although in some cases, it may be detached from the bodies of the axis and C3 [7]. There is a double mechanism of injury. Initially, a hyperextension force will fracture the pars interarticular without any serious ligamentous injury. Then, a flexion-compression force will rupture the posterior longitudinal ligament and the intervertebral disc, resulting in anterior dislocation of the body of the axis and varying degrees of angulation. Type III (4 %) results from flexion-compression and is characterized by bilateral fractures of the pars interarticularis and unilateral or bilateral dislocation of the C2–C3 facet joints, and significant anterior dislocation and angulation of the axis (Fig. 8.6). This type of injury is considered particularly unstable because of the free floating articular processes, and it is most commonly associated with neurological deficits [7].

In 1985, Levine and Edwards modified Effendi's classification by adding one subtype: type IIa results from combined flexion-distraction and is characterized by increased anterior angulation of the body of the axis without anterior dislocation (Fig. 8.7). These fractures are considered unstable [5]. Francis et al. classification [3] includes five types as follows:

Type I, anterior displacement <3.5 mm and angulation <11°.

Type II, anterior displacement <3.5 mm and angulation >11°.

Type III, anterior displacement >3.5 mm but less than half the width of C3 and angulation <11°.

Type IV, displacement >3.5 mm but less than half the width of C3 and angulation >11°.

Type V, associated rupture of the intervertebral disc.

The first two classifications have been shown to be more realistic and are accepted by the majority of orthopaedic surgeons.

The clinical presentation of the traumatic spondylolisthesis of the axis is relatively mild. There is restriction of rotational movements and

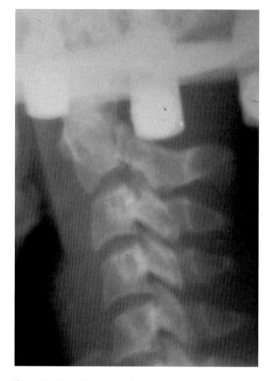

Fig. 8.7 Type IIa traumatic spondylolisthesis in a halo vest

local pain. Neurological deficits are uncommon and are usually caused by a double level injury of the spine, most commonly the atlas, due to the development of a higher degree of instability of the upper cervical spine. The neurological injury may be the result of direct injury of the spinal cord

or the vertebral arteries, or it can be caused with an attempt to reduce the fracture. It can be mild, with paresthesia, or more severe with hemiparesis, hemiplegia and Brown-Sequard syndrome. Arnold type cervical pain is uncommon. Most often, it is transient and subsides with appropriate treatment. In 79 % of cases, there is a coexistent injury to the head or to another level of the spinal cord. In 30 % of cases, a fracture of the arch or an avulsion fracture of the body of the axis or C3 may coexist (Fig. 8.8a). The most common associated injury is the fracture of the posterior arch of the atlas. Fractures of the lower cervical, thoracic or lumbar spine may also occur (Fig. 8.8b) [8, 9].

In 90 % of cases, the diagnosis is based on standard radiographs. Computed tomography may provide additional information on the extent and nature of the fracture. If the fracture line extents to the transverse foramen then angiography is essential to assess the vertebral arteries (Fig. 8.9). The ligamentous injuries are better evaluated by magnetic resonance imaging.

Although the fracture line involves the pars interarticularis bilaterally, most of the times, this is not in a symmetrical manner due to the different combinations of rotational forces that participate each time to the mechanism of injury (Fig. 8.10). The presence of fracture asymmetry implies the rotational deformation of the axis and thus could render closed reduction through skeletal traction problematic and probably

Fig. 8.8 a. Traumatic spondylolisthesis (type I) combined with a tear drop fracture of the axis. **b**. Traumatic spondylolisthesis with concomitant fracture of C5 (Courtesy of Dr. Zachariou)

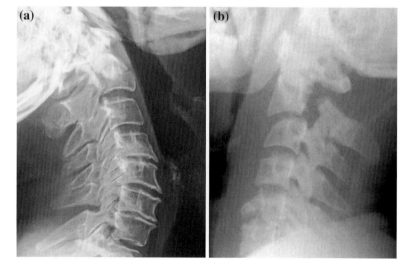

(a)   (b)

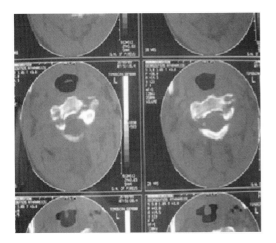

Fig. 8.9 Traumatic spondylolisthesis. Reconstruction image at the level of C2; the slice is sowing extension of the fracture to the left transverse foramen threatening the vertebral artery

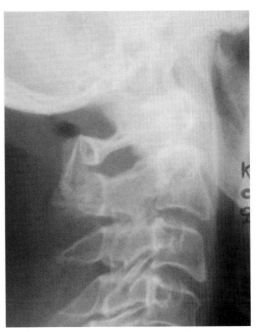

Fig. 8.11 Brook's technique with nylon sutures

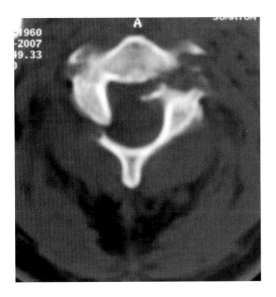

Fig. 8.10 Asymmetry of fractures (Courtesy of Dr. Zachariou)

insufficient. Moreover, if the fracture line extends to the transverse foramen, the vertebral artery may be injured during skeletal traction [6]. The asymmetrical fractures may have an increased incidence of pseudarthrosis due to their increased degree of instability. However, it seems that this is not true, as recent studies did not show any relation between fracture asymmetry and outcome [10].

Traumatic spondylolisthesis of the axis is generally considered as a stable injury if no injuries to the C2–C3 intervertebral disc, the posterior longitudinal ligament or the articular surfaces are present. The criteria of instability, as defined by White and Panjabi [11] and Roy Camille et al. [12], involve anterior dislocation of >3−5 mm and angulation >11°. In addition, Coric et al. [13] suggested that an anterior dislocation of >6 mm or displacement of the body >2 mm in dynamic radiographs should be considered as additional signs of instability. Type IIa and certainly type III are unstable injuries.

Once the injury has been recognized and classified, proper treatment should begin. The aim of treatment is the anatomic reduction and proper stabilization of the fracture. Initially, type I fractures should be treated conservatively with immobilization with a Philadelphia collar or a halo vest for 8–10 weeks. If following dynamic flexion and extension radiographs instability is present, operative treatment is indicated. Type II fractures require closed reduction with skeletal traction and extension of the cervical spine. This is achieved by placing a pillow between the

Fig. 8.12 a. Type III traumatic spondylolisthesis, **b**. Two years after the injury, spontaneous C2–C3 fusion is observed

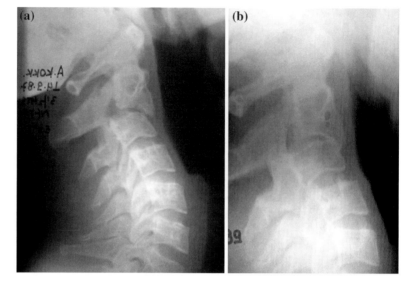

scapulae of the patient. Five to seven days later, the traction is removed. If reduction of the fracture is acceptable (anterior dislocation <4–5 mm and angulation <10°), a halo vest should be applied for 3 months. If there is loss of reduction, skeletal traction must be continued for 4–6 weeks followed by a halo vest for another 6 weeks. Type IIa fractures are reduced through extension of the cervical spine combined with mild axial compression. In this type of injury, operative treatment is indicated. Skeletal traction should not be applied because the back sliding of the intervertebral disc causes widening of the posterior intervertebral space and kyphotic deformity of the cervical spine. Type III fractures should be treated initially with traction through a halo vest; however, proper reduction is not always possible. Surgical treatment is strongly advocated [5, 14–16] as reduction in the dislocated fracture is feasible only through surgical intervention since the inferior articular facets have been separated from the rest of the axis and cannot be reduced by ligamentotaxis. Posterior C2–C3 stabilization is recommended and will also result in correction of the kyphotic deformity. Anterior stabilization should be avoided although it is advocated [17], because of the injury of the anterior longitudinal ligament that is the only remaining stabilizing structure. Furthermore,

anterior stabilization should also be avoided if there is an avulsion fracture at the anterior-inferior angle of the body of the axis. Alternatively, the spinous processes of the axis and C3 can be stabilized with wires [18], or other techniques (Fig. 8.11) [5, 19–22]. Important to note is the fact that nearly 80% of cases of traumatic spondylolisthesis, despite the type of injury, spontaneous fusion, mainly anteriorly, between the bodies of the axis and C3 may occur (Fig. 8.12a, b) [5, 9]. In case of failure to reduce the fracture, surgery via an anterior [17] or posterior [23] approach is indicated.

8.2 Results

Literature data report that most of the patients with traumatic spondylolisthesis of the axis can be treated successfully conservatively [9, 13, 24, 25]. However, there are studies pointing out to surgical stabilization due to the instability of these injuries [26]. Mestdagh et al. [27] observed greater range of motion of the cervical spine in 30 patients treated conservatively with halo vest than in 11 patients who were treated surgically. They recommended that initial treatment in every patient should be conservative unless there is evident instability or pseudarthrosis of the fracture. Grady et al. [28] treated 16 patients with halo vest, eight patients with Philadelphia collar and three patients with bed rest. Fracture healing was achieved in all their patients, and the authors claimed that the Philadelphia collar and the halo vest have comparable results in the treatment of the minimally displaced fractures. We share the same opinion provided to properly apply the conservative treatment; this may require a prolonged absence of the patients from their everyday activities.

References

1. Haughton S (1866) On hanging considered from a mechanical and physiological point of view. London, Edinburg and Dublin philosophical magazine and journal of science 4th series 1866 32:23–34
2. Garber JN (1964) Abnormalities of the atlas and axis vertebra—congenital and traumatic. J Bone Jt Surg Am 46-Á:1782–1791
3. Francis W, Fielding W, Hawkins R, Pepin J, Hensinger R (1981) Traumatic spondylolisthesis of the axis. J Bone Jt Surg Br 63-B:313–318
4. Effendi B, Roy D, Cornish B, Dussault RG, Laurin CA. (1981) Fractures of the ring of the axis. A classification based on the analysis of 131 cases. J Bone Jt Surg Br 63-B:319–327
5. Levine A, Edwards C (1985) The management of traumatic Spondylolisthesis of the axis. J Bone Jt Surg Am 67:217–226
6. Junge A, El-Sheik M, Celik I, Gotzen L (2002) Pathomorphology, diagnosis and treatment of "hangman's fractures". Unfallchirurg 105:775–782
7. Moon MS, Moon JL, Moon YW, Sun DH, Choi WT (2001) Traumatic spondylolisthesis of the axis: forty two cases. Bull Hosp Jt Dis 60:61–66
8. Morel E, Ilharreborde B, Zadegan F, Rillardon L, Guigui P (2009) An unusual hangman's fracture: description and surgical management. Orthop Traumatol Surg Res 95(3):229–233
9. Korres DS (1999) The cervical spine. Traumatology and pathology. By Litsas Medical Editions. Athens
10. Samaha C, Laennec JY, Laport C, Saillant G. (2000) Hangman's fracture: The relationship between asymmetry and instability. J Bone Joint Surg Br 82:1046–1052
11. White HI, Panjabi M (1990) Clinical biomechanics of spine. In: Lippincott (ed) Spine injuries. Philadelphia, 146.154
12. Roy-Camille R, Bleunie JF, Saillant G, Judet T (1979) Fractures de l'odontoïde associée à une fracture des pédicules de l'axis. Rev Chir Orthop 65:387–391
13. Coric D, Wilson JA, Kelly DL Jr (1996) Treatment of traumatic spondylolisthesis of the axis with nonrigid immobilization: a review of 64 cases. J Neurosurg 85:55–554
14. American Association of Neurological Surgeons (2002) Isolated Fractures of the Axis in adults. Neurosurg 50(Suppl 3):105–147
15. Boullosa JLR, Colli BO, Carlotti CG (2004). Surgical management of axis' traumatic spondylolisthesis. Arq Neuropsiquiatr 62(3-B): 821–826
16. Barros TE, Bohlaman HH, Capen DA, Cotler J, Dons K, Bierring-Sorensen F, Marchesi DG, Zigler JE (1999) Traumatic spondylolisthesis of the axis: analysis of Management. Spinal Cord 37:166–171
17. Tuite GF, Papadopoulos SM, Sonntag VK (1992) Gaspar plate fixation for the treatment of complex hangman's fractures. Neurosurgery 30(5):761–764
18. Brooks AL, Jenkins EB (1978) Atlanto-axial arthrodesis by the wedge compression method. J Bone Joint Surg 60-A(3):279–284
19. Harms J, Melcher RP (2001) Posterior C1–C2 fusion with polyaxial screw and rod fixation. Spine 26: 2467–2471
20. Ying Z, Yuan W, Wang X et al (2008) Anterior cervical discectomy and fusion for unstable traumatic spondylolisthesis of the axis. Spine 33(3):255–258
21. Sugimoto Y, Ito Y, Shimokawa T, Shiozaki Y, Mazaki T (2010) Percutaneous screw fixation for traumatic spondylolisthesis of the axis using iso-C3D fluoroscopy- assisted navigation (case report). Minim Invasive Neurosurg 53(2):83–85
22. Barnechi G (2008) Traumatologia vertebrale. Chap7: fratture dell' epistrofeo pp 127–162
23. Tian W, Weng C, Liu B et al (2011) Posterior fixation and fusion of unstable hangman fracture by using intraoperative three-dimensional fluoroscopy-based Navigation. Eur Spine J (online, November 2011)
24. Muller EJ, Wick M, Muhr G (2000) Traumatic spondylolisthesis of the Axis: Treatment rationale based on the stability of the different fracture types. Eur Spine J 9:123–128
25. Ranieri A, Domenicucci M, Landi A, Rastelli E, Raco A (2011) Conservative treatment of neural arch fractures of the axis: computed tomography scan and x-ray study on consolidation time. World Neurosurg 75(2):314–319
26. Cornish L (1968) Traumatic spondylolisthesis of the axis. J Bone Jt Surg Br 50:31–43
27. Mestdagh H, Letendart J, Sensey JJ, Duquennoy A (1984) Treatment of fractures of the posterior axial arch. Results of 41 cases. Rev Chir Orthop Reparatrice Appar Mot 70:21–28
28. Grady MS, Howard MA, Jane JA, Persing JA (1986) Use of the Philadelphia collar as an alternative to the halo vest in patients with C-2, C-3 fractures. Neurosurgery 18:151–156

Multiple or Complex Fractures

9

Demetrios S. Korres and Andreas F. Mavrogenis

Multiple or complex fractures of the axis are rare injuries occurring following the application, nearly simultaneously, of more than one forces; hyperextension seem to be the predominant force [1, 2]. This injury was reported in the past but not as a separated entity [3] and a low attention has been given to it. In line with the literature, the incidence in our experience was 0.9 % of all cervical spine fractures or 5 % of all axis fractures [1–4]. The diagnosis of these injuries depends on the precise history of the accident's conditions, a high degree of suspicion and careful imaging examination. The clinical examination reveals the same findings as in isolated lesions (such as odontoid process fracture or traumatic spondylolisthesis) that is pain on the neck and the occiput, painful and severe restriction of the range of motion of the cervical spine, and a higher incidence of neurological signs because of greater displacement and related instability.

Radiographs should include the lateral (Fig. 9.1a) and open mouth views, while CT-Scan should follow in order to better visualize the injured area; here to note the need for acquisition of <1 mm thin slice width and the importance for acquisition of reconstructive images or even 3-D reconstruction (Fig. 9.1b, c).

The combination of two fractures concerning a traumatic spondylolisthesis and a fracture of the odontoid process is the commonest type of injury [2, 5], while other combinations include a tear drop fracture to a traumatic spondylolisthesis, fracture of the odontoid process with an associated fracture of the lateral mass (Figs. 9.2) [6], or very rarely simultaneous fractures of all three anatomic elements of the axis (Fig. 9.1a) [2].

The treatment depends on the stability of the injury. Stable fractures are better treated conservatively with initial immobilization using either skeletal traction or a halo vest for a period of 10–12 weeks, and a promising prognosis. Unstable lesions are treated surgically depending on the unstable level. However, not always, is better for the patients to offer the best opportunity with a less aggressive surgery. So, in some instances, it will be worthy to operate only the more unstable injury for example only an unstable fracture of the odontoid process and treat conservatively a type I traumatic spondylolisthesis or a tear drop fracture.

Initially the fracture has to be reduced by skeletal traction or in halo, and then stabilized using either a modified Brooks technique [3], or osteosynthesis with screws and plates or even

D. S. Korres (✉)
3rd Orthopaedic Department, KAT Hospital,
University of Athens, Heyden 10, 104 34, Athens,
Attika, Greece
e-mail: demiskorres@gmail.com

A. F. Mavrogenis
First Department of Orthopaedics, University of
Athens, Attikon University Hospital, 41 Ventouri,
155 62, Athens, Attika, Greece
e-mail: afm@otenet.gr

D. S. Korres (ed.), *The Axis Vertebra*,
DOI: 10.1007/978-88-470-5232-1_9, © Springer-Verlag Italia 2013

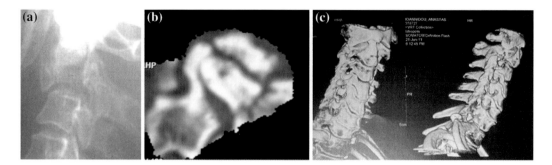

Fig. 9.1 Multiple fractures of the axis. **a** Lateral radiograph shows a tear drop fracture, traumatic spondylolisthesis and fracture of the odontoid process. **b** Reconstruction image shows a double fracture of the odontoid process. **c** 3-D CT scan reconstruction shows a tear drop fracture (*white arrow*) and traumatic spondylolisthesis (*black arrow*)

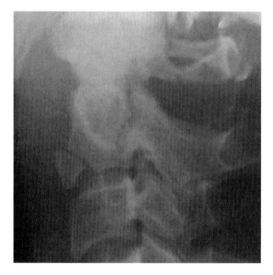

Fig. 9.2 Tear drop fracture and traumatic spondylolisthesis associated with a fracture of the posterior arch of the atlas

The management of all the previously described injuries either conservative or operative should be completed with an individualized program of physical therapy. In the post-injury, and more important the post-operative period all cases have to be rehabilitated appropriately and with care. The soft tissue injury, fractures and particular fusion in anatomic position will influence the biomechanics of the occipito-cervical area.

with anterior screw fixation of the odontoid process and posterior fusion [2, 7, 8]. Posterior fusion, although it has a high rate of success it is not without problems regarding the function of the cervical spine as it reduces significant the range of motion in rotation and flexion–extension [9]. The lack in the literature of large series is probably the reason why there is not a clear consensus regarding the management of these injuries, thus, it is not possible to easily treat these so vary lesions.

References

1. Korres DS, Papagelopoulos PJ, Mavrogenis AF, Sapkas GS, Patsinevelos A, Kyriazopoulos P, Evangelopoulos D (2004) Multiple fractures of the axis. Orthopedics 27:1096–1099
2. Roy-Camille R, Lafosse L, Bouchet TH, Judet TH (1986) Les associations traumatiques du rachis cervical superieur. In: Rachis cervical superieur, Masson Paris, pp 137–141
3. Burke JT, Harris JH Jr (1989) Acute injuries of the axis vertebra. Skeletal Radiol 8:335–346
4. Gleizes V, Jacquot FP, Signoret F, Feron JM (2000) Combined injuries in the upper cervical spine: clinical and epidemiological data over a 14 years period. Eur Spine J 9:386–392
5. Roy-Camille R, Bleunie JF, Saillant G, Judet T (1979) Fractures de l'odontoid associée à une fracture des pédicules de l'axis. Rev Chir Orthop 65:387–391
6. Signoret F, Feron JM, Bonfait H, Patel A (1986) Fractured odontoid with fractured superior articular process of the axis. J Bone Jt Surg 68-B:182–184
7. Blondel B, Metellus PH, Fuentes S, Duterte G, Dufour H (2009) Single anterior procedure for stabilization of

a three-part fracture of the axis (odontoid and hang-man fracture). Spine 34(7):E255–E257

8. Koller H, Assuncao A, Kammermeier V et al (2006) Simultaneous anterior arthrodesis C2–C3 and anterior odontoid screw fixation for stabilization of a 4-part fracture of the axis: a technical description. J Spinal Disord Tech 19:362–367

9. Apfelbaum RI, Lonser RR, Veres R et al (2000) Direct anterior screw fixation for recent and remote odontoid fractures. J Neurosurg 93:227–236

Atlantoaxial Dislocation

10

Panagiotis K. Karampinas and Demetrios S. Korres

The atlantoaxial joint is the most mobile segment of the spine. It allows 3 planes of movement: angular motion (flexion and extension), rotation (right and left) and linear motion, translation (anterior and posterior, right and left). Four are the types of atlantoaxial dislocation: anteroposterior dislocation, rotatory dislocation, central or vertical dislocation and mixed dislocation (any two or three of the above) (Fig. 10.1). Anteroposterior dislocation is in one plane and one direction, due to transverse ligament laxity and when there is os odontoideum. Central-vertical instability is characterized by dislocation of the body of the axis into the ring of the atlas and should be differentiated from basilar invagination that is upwards (vertical) displacement of the atlas. The rotatory dislocation is usually in one plane and one direction [1–3]. Atlantoaxial rotatory dislocation (AARD) was first described by Bell in 1830 and is characterized by rotational displacement between the atlas and the axis [4].

10.1 Atlantoaxial Rotatory Dislocation

10.1.1 Etiology and Anatomy

The atlantoaxial stability depends on ligamentous integrity and joint's anatomical elements (articular surface and joint capsule). It is a rare injury in children and even more rare in adult. It is often encountered in young patients (0.6 %) [5–7]. Children are characterized by greater ligamentous laxity and wider range of joint motion (horizontal orientation of the articular surface). Therefore, higher forces are required to provoque ligamentous injuries that would result in joint dislocation [1, 5, 6, 8].

Atlantoaxial rotatory dislocation may result either primarily from osseous or ligamentous abnormality after direct trauma or secondary to other entities such as congenital cervical spine anomalies, degenerative rheumatoid arthritis (Grisel's syndrome), and more rarely tumors and spinal infections. Congenital pathologies include Down's (symptomatic 1–2 % and asymptomatic 10–20 %), Morquio's and Marfan's syndromes [4, 5, 9, 10]. Trauma alone is a rare cause of atlantoaxial joint rotatory dislocation and if so it is probably associated with other injuries of the lower levels of the spine. The traumatic cause of atlantoaxial dislocation may coexist with those pathologic entities. Conditions with associated laxity carry an increased incidence of traumatic atlantoaxial dislocation [1, 7, 11, 12].

P. K. Karampinas (✉) · D. S. Korres
3rd Orthopaedic Department, KAT Hospital,
University of Athens, Nikis 2, 14561, Athens,
Attika, Greece
e-mail: karapana@yahoo.com

D. S. Korres (ed.), *The Axis Vertebra*,
DOI: 10.1007/978-88-470-5232-1_10, © Springer-Verlag Italia 2013

The transverse ligament contributes to the atlantoaxial joint stability by stabilizing atlas in the anteroposterior line. At the second line of defense there are the alar ligaments which prevent the anterior shift of the atlas and the excessive rotation of the atlantoaxial joint. Biomechanical studies evaluating the transverse ligament concluded that it allows 65° of rotation of the atlas around the odontoid apex thus stabilizing the atlas in the anteroposterior plane. Complete or contralateral atlantoaxial dislocation with obliteration of the spine canal (>12 mm) can be consider safe when transverse ligament tear and anterior sliding of the atlas <5 mm in children and 3 mm in adults or rotation >45° are observed. Alar ligaments are considered as rotational stabilizers and their tears are responsible for rotational dislocation. Mechanisms associated with atlantoaxial dislocation include flexion-extension, distraction as well as rotational forces [1, 5, 12, 13].

10.1.2 Classification

AARD is classified according to Fielding and Hawkins (Fig. 10.1) [14]. Type I injuries are characterized by rotation of atlas associated with bilateral dislocation but without sliding in the anteroposterior plane. In Type II injuries, an anteroposterior sliding of the atlas not more than 3–5 mm with associated contralateral dislocation is observed (rotationally unstable injury with incompetence of the transverse alar ligament). Type III injuries are characterized by sliding of atlas in the anteroposterior plane >5 mm and bilateral dislocation (unstable injury with transverse and alar ligament tear), while Type IV injuries show posterior sliding of the atlas with associated dislocation of one or both atlantoaxial joints (unstable rare injury associated with congenital aplasia of odontoid apex). Apart those types, a vertically upwards dislocation may be encounter, although it represents a rare lesion [15]. Type I injury is the most common type, rotationally unstable but with intact transverse ligament, while type IV is rare but potentially dangerous [16].

10.1.3 Clinical Presentation and Differential Diagnosis

The patient with AARD usually presents with torticollis, distortion of the head in anterolateral flexion toward the injured site and rotation toward the opposite site. Torticollis is subdivided according to the etiology in traumatic and non traumatic. Traumatic torticollis is recognized after rotatory atlantoaxial dislocation, atlantoaxial subluxation, cervical spine fracture, muscular and ligamentous injures. Differential diagnosis should also include congenital torticollis, infections of the spine (otitis media, pharyngitis or retropharyngeal abscess), cervical adenitis and tumors. Traumatic torticollis should always raise suspicions to the Emergency Room Physicians to evaluate this type of injuries. On clinical examination head and facial injuries may be present. Other useful clinical signs include: (a) sternocleidomastoid muscle contraction contralateral to the injury in a effort to reduce head distortion, (b) difficulty to bring the head back to the middle line, (c) limited range of motion of the cervical spine and (d) severe pain while attempting the reduction of the distortion [6–8, 13, 17].

AARD can be often misdiagnosed. Such injury can be easily reduced if recognized and treated within the first few hours (no later than 24 h). Delayed treatment of unstable atlantoaxial dislocation causes stiffness of the atlantoaxial joints due to muscle, capsule and ligament shrinking after repeated micro-dislocations and inflammations. Moreover, voice alteration, due to pressure on the laryngeal nerve and the vocal cords, difficulty in swallowing and displacement of the shoulder can also be observed. Lower cranial nerve palsies, myelopathy and injury of the cervical artery have been reported following unstable AARD. The clinical picture of these injuries varies according to the severity of the spinal cord injury and can even cause death. Symptomatic patients have higher risk of progressive neurological symptoms, sensory deficit, neurogenic bladder, upper motor neuron signs, hemiplegia and quadriplegia [6–8, 18].

Fig. 10.1 Schematic presentation of Fielding's and Hawkin's classification for atlantoaxial instability

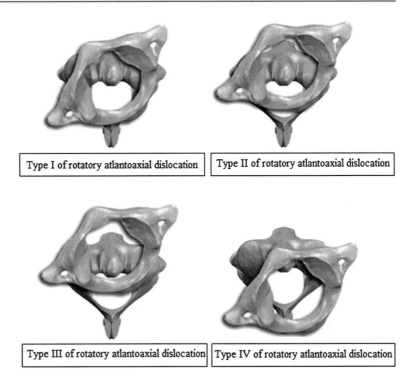

| Type I of rotatory atlantoaxial dislocation | Type II of rotatory atlantoaxial dislocation |

| Type III of rotatory atlantoaxial dislocation | Type IV of rotatory atlantoaxial dislocation |

10.1.4 Radiographic Evaluation

The radiographic evaluation is difficult due to the injury's nature and the technically demanding appropriate radiographs. Evaluation of traumatic cases should be performed immediately and include the entire cervical column, particularly in patients with a Glasgow Coma Scale of <13 (C1-T1). For non-traumatic cases, evaluation can take place even after a week of conservative treatment with cervical collar and anti-inflammatory medication. Radiographs should include anteroposterior, lateral and open-mouth odontoid plane views (Fig. 10.2), while potential instability can be identified on dynamic flexion-extension views. The evaluation of the entire cervical spine even up to T1 vertebra or lower is mandatory to rule out double level injures of the spine [17].

The open-mouth odontoid view can be indicative in detecting potential asymmetry between the atlas and axis with unilateral displacement of the lateral mass and diastasis of the atlanto-odontoid space. During traumatic torticollis, suspicion of rotatory dislocation must be set when the distance between the odontoid apex and atlas [atlanto–dens interval (ADI)] is >5 mm and an anterior sliding of the atlas with discontinuity of the posterior cervical line is present (Fig. 10.3). Prevertebral swelling (>7 mm) at this level, is an important radiological finding for upper cervical spine trauma. This injury shows a high risk for neurological damage. The posterior atlanto–dens interval (PADI), the available space for the spinal cord between the posterior border of the dens and the anterior border of the posterior tubercle, has to be >14 mm. A PADI <12 mm is associated with an increased risk of neurological damage [6, 7, 11, 19]. If radiological examination cannot be conclusive, a CT-scan should be performed (Fig. 10.4). The three dimensional reconstruction CT-scan provides an accurate picture of the injury and its severity (Fig. 10.5). In certain cases, a dynamic CT-scan can also be performed [20, 21]. Villas et al. [22] correlated the severity of injury with

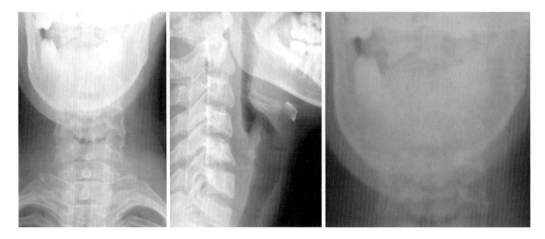

Fig. 10.2 Anteroposterior, lateral and open-mouth views of the cervical spine show a type I traumatic rotatory atlantoaxial dislocation

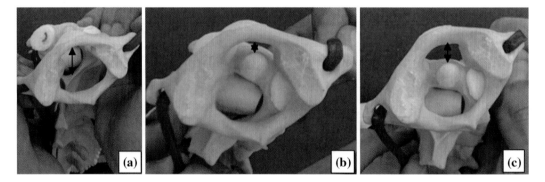

Fig. 10.3 The posterior atlanto–dens interval and atlanto–dens interval. The PADI has to be >14 mm (**a**). The ADI is >3 mm (**b**) and 5 mm (**c**) during rotatory unstable traumatic dislocation suspicion

Fig. 10.4 CT scans show
a type I traumatic rotatory
atlantoaxial dislocation

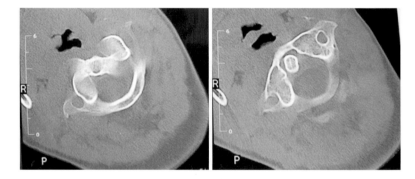

the percentage of the uncovered joint surface following dislocation. Additionally, MRI represents a reliable tool for the detection of transverse and alar ligament lesions [6, 7, 16, 23, 24].

10.1.5 Treatment

Treatment must start immediately after the injury to avoid shrinking of the soft tissue of the joints and stiffness of the deformed cervical

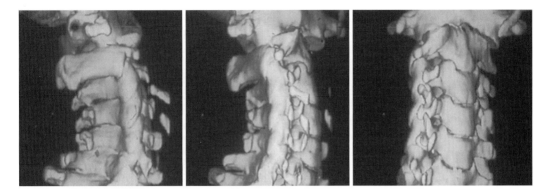

Fig. 10.5 Three dimensional reconstruction CT scans show a type I traumatic AARD

spine. The time elapsed between diagnosis and treatment determines the results and prognosis. Treatment time has been shown to correlate with the recurrence of dislocation recurrence and failure of reduction. After the diagnosis of atlantoaxial dislocation with a CT-scan, reduction must be attempted with manipulation and application of jaw-occipital or skeletal traction.

Reduction of the dislocation has to be accomplished within the first 2–3 days following the injury [6, 7, 17]. Following adequate reduction, patient's cervical spine is immobilized with a cervical collar or a halo vest for 6–10 weeks. The patient should be followed up regularly with radiographs until stability of the cervical spine is achieved. Treatment with closed reduction and immobilization resolves the torticollis and restores the distortion in almost 95% of cases. Patients receiving delayed treatment require cervical skeletal traction for 5–8 days and immobilization for a longer period, until 3 months with a halo vest. If the time elapsed between diagnosis and treatment is more than 3 weeks, a high rate of reduction failure and if reduced (difficult) recurrence is observed [6–8, 11–13, 18].

When the treatment is delayed or the dislocation is not reduced, permanent deformity is installed making impossible the reduction of the lesion. In such cases, reduction with a hallo vest or surgical treatment and arthrodesis of the atlantoaxial complex to avoid further instability represents the only feasible treatment options (Fig. 10.6).

The described surgical techniques include Brook's and Gallie's sublaminar wiring technique, Magerl's transarticular screw fusion, as well other less often applied techniques [25, 26].

Fig. 10.6 Schematic presentation and radiograph show an unstable type IV traumatic rotatory atlantoaxial dislocation

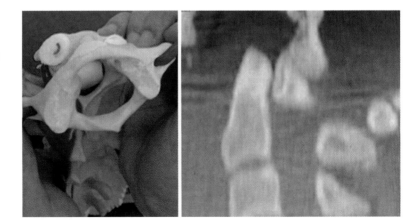

Posterior fusion with transarticular screw fixation and sublaminar wiring is the most stable treatment technique [27]. The surgical intervention cannot fully restore rotational deformity of the cervical spine and achieve a normal function of the atlantoaxial area. Main goals of the surgical treatment are to protect the spinal cord, stabilize the spinal column, decompress neural tissue and reduce the deformity. The functional and range of motion deficit are compensated by the lower cervical spine [6, 8, 16, 28–31].

References

1. White AA 3rd, Panjabi MM (1978) The clinical biomechanics of the occipitoatlantoaxial complex. Orthop Clin North Am 9(4):867–878
2. Goel A, Bhatjiwale M, Desai K (1998) Basilar invagination: a study based on 190 surgically treated patients. J Neurosurg 88(6):962–968. doi: 10.3171/jns.1998.88.6.0962
3. Tulsi RS (1978) Some specific anatomical features of the atlas and axis: dens, epitransverse process and articular facets. Aust N Z J Surg 48(5):570–574
4. Greenberg AD (1968) Atlanto-axial dislocations. Brain 91(4):655–684
5. Swischuk LE (1977) Anterior displacement of C2 in children: physiologic or pathologic. Radiology 122(3):759–763
6. Subach BR, McLaughlin MR, Albright AL, Pollack IF (1998) Current management of pediatric atlantoaxial rotatory subluxation. Spine (Phila Pa 1976) 23(20):2174–2179
7. Crook TB, Eynon CA (2005) Traumatic atlantoaxial rotatory subluxation. Emerg Med J 22(9):671–672. doi:10.1136/emj.2003.013045
8. Maile S, Slongo T (2007) Atlantoaxial rotatory subluxation: realignment and discharge within 48 h. Eur J Emerg Med 14(3):167–169. doi: 10.1097/MEJ.0b013e328014081c
9. Morton RE, Khan MA, Murray-Leslie C, Elliott S (1995) Atlantoaxial instability in down's syndrome: a five year follow up study. Arch Dis Child 72 (2):115–118; Discussion 118–119
10. Muniz AE, Belfer RA (1999) Atlantoaxial rotary subluxation in children. Pediatr Emerg Care 15(1):25–29
11. Schwarz N (1998) The fate of missed atlanto-axial rotatory subluxation in children. Arch Orthop Trauma Surg 117(4–5):288–289
12. Moore KR, Frank EH (1995) Traumatic atlantoaxial rotatory subluxation and dislocation. Spine (Phila Pa 1976) 20(17):1928–1930
13. Niibayashi H (1998) Atlantoaxial rotatory dislocation: a case report. Spine (Phila Pa 1976) 23(13):1494–1496
14. Fielding JW, Hawkins RJ (1977) Atlanto-axial rotatory fixation (fixed rotatory subluxation of the atlanto-axial joint). J Bone Joint Surg Am 59(1):37–44
15. Payer M, Wetzel S, Kelekis A, Jenny B (2005) Traumatic vertical atlantoaxial dislocation. J Clin Neurosci 12(6):704–706
16. Yoon DH, Yang KH, Kim KN, Oh SH (2003) Posterior atlanto-axial dislocation without fracture. J Neurosurg 98(1):73–76
17. Phillips WA, Hensinger RN (1989) The management of rotatory atlanto-axial subluxation in children. J Bone Joint Surg Am 71(5):664–668
18. Govender S, Kumar KP (2002) Staged reduction and stabilisation in chronic atlantoaxial rotatory fixation. J Bone Joint Surg Br 84(5):727–731
19. Gallie WE (1937) Skeletal traction in the treatment of fractures and dislocations of the cervical spine. Ann Surg 106(4):770–776
20. Rinaldi I, Mullins WJ Jr, Delaney WF, Fitzer PM, Tornberg DN (1979) Computerized tomographic demonstration of rotational atlanto-axial fixation. J Neurosurg 50(1):115–119. doi:10.3171/jns.1979. 50.1.0115
21. Pratt H, Davies E, King L (2008) Traumatic injuries of the c1/c2 complex: computed tomographic imaging appearances. Curr Probl Diagn Radiol 37(1):26–38. doi:10.1067/j.cpradiol.2007.07.001
22. Villas C, Arriagada C, Zubieta JL (1999) Preliminary CT study of C1-C2 rotational mobility in normal subjects. Eur Spine J 8(3):223–228
23. Willauschus WG, Kladny B, Beyer WF, Gluckert K, Arnold H, Scheithauer R (1995) Lesions of the alar ligaments: in vivo and in vitro studies with magnetic resonance imaging. Spine (Phila Pa 1976) 20(23): 2493–2498
24. Woodring JH, Lee C (1992) The role and limitations of computed tomographic scanning in the evaluation of cervical trauma. J Trauma 33(5):698–708
25. Harms J, Melcher RP (2001) Posterior C1-C2 fusion with polyaxial screw and rod fixation. Spine (Phila Pa 1976) 26(22):2467–2471
26. Du Toit G (1976) Lateral atlanto-axial arthrodesis: a screw fixation technique. S Afr J Surg 14(1):9–12
27. Grob D, Crisco JJ 3rd, Panjabi MM, Wang P, Dvorak J (1992) Biomechanical evaluation of four different posterior atlantoaxial fixation techniques. Spine 17(5):480–490
28. Haid RW Jr, Subach BR, McLaughlin MR, Rodts GE, Jr, Wahlig JB, Jr (2001) C1-C2 transarticular screw fixation for atlantoaxial instability: a 6 year experience. Neurosurgery 49(1):65–68; Discussion 69–70
29. Lee SH, Kim ES, Sung JK, Park YM, Eoh W (2010) Clinical and radiological comparison of treatment of atlantoaxial instability by posterior C1-C2

transarticular screw fixation or C1 lateral mass-C2 pedicle screw fixation. J Clin Neurosci 17(7): 886–892. doi:10.1016/j.jocn.2009.10.008

30. Li WL, Chi YL, Xu HZ, Wang XY, Lin Y, Huang QS, Mao FM (2010) Percutaneous anterior transarticular screw fixation for atlantoaxial instability: a case series. J Bone Joint Surg Br 92(4):545–549. doi:10. 1302/0301-620X.92B4.22790

31. Elgafy H, Potluri T, Goel VK, Foster S, Faizan A, Kulkarni N (2010) Biomechanical analysis comparing three C1-C2 transarticular screw salvaging fixation techniques. Spine (Phila Pa 1976) 35(4):378–385. doi: 10.1097/BRS.0b013e3181bc9cb5

Part III

Surgical Approaches

11

Andrea Angelini and Roberto Casadei

In 1954, Lahey used an anterior approach between the carotid sheath and the esophagus anterior to the sternocleidomastoid muscle [1]. In 1957, Southwick provided a more detailed description of the fascial planes traversed in this surgery [2] and Robinson in 1959 performed the first anterolateral retropharyngeal procedure [3]. In the past, anterior approach to the upper cervical spine have requested a transoral approach [4], a lateral extra pharyngeal approach [5], a dislocation of the temporal mandibular joint [6], an osteotomy of the mandible and a tongue splitting approach [7]. Surgical exposure of the upper cervical spine is considered difficult and dangerous because of the anatomical complexity, the deep location, and the proximity to vital neurovascular structures. These approaches to the spine generally are performed by an experienced spine surgeon and, as a rule, this type of surgery is not appropriate for those who only occasionally perform spinal surgeries. A team approach is preferred to use the skill of an orthopaedic surgeon, a neurosurgeon, a thoracic surgeon and a head and neck surgeon. Orthopaedic surgeons should have a working knowledge of the underlying viscera. Anterior spine surgery has few complications, but a high risk of significant morbidity. Thus these approaches should be used with care and only in appropriate patients. The choice of the approach which would be performed depends on the preference and the experience of the surgeon, the patient's age and medical condition, the segment of the spine involved, the underlying pathology and the presence or absence of neural compression.

The surgical approach to the upper cervical spine (C1–C2) can be (Fig. 11.1):

1. Anterior, with transoral approach and its modifications,
2. Lateral,
3. Anterolateral,
4. Posterior, with the direct approach to the posterior arch of the atlas and axis.

11.1 Anterior (Transoral) Approach

Contra-indications for the anterior transoral approach include elderly patients with rheumatoid arthritis, patients with mandibular disorders, and those with large tumors with vertebral artery involvement.

Preoperative planning should include evaluation of medical comorbidities and nutritional status, dental and oral cavity evaluation for infection, and administration of standard preoperative antibiotic therapy with an intravenous cephalosporin and metronidazole.

A. Angelini (✉) R. Casadei
Department of Orthopaedics, University of Bologna,
Istituto Ortopedico Rizzoli, Via Pupilli 1, 40136,
Bologna, Italy
e-mail: andrea.angelini@ior.it

R. Casadei
e-mail: roberto.casadei@ior.it

D. S. Korres (ed.), *The Axis Vertebra*,
DOI: 10.1007/978-88-470-5232-1_11, © Springer-Verlag Italia 2013

Fig. 11.1 Cross section at the level of the axis. Note the surgical approaches to the axis. *m* muscle, *v* vein

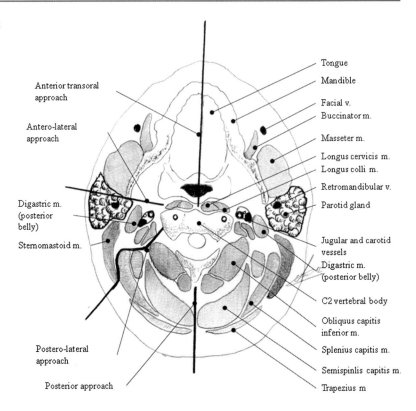

11.1.1 Position

The patient is placed in a supine position with the head in a padded headrest. Nasotracheal intubation is preferred. The lips and tongue are coated with 5 % cortisone cream. The oropharyngeal area is prepared with antiseptic solution (povidone iodine), and a throat packing is placed to prevent debris from falling into dependent laryngeal spaces or the trachea. An epinephrine solution is injected along the site of planned incision. The patient can also be placed in a mild reverse-Trendelenburg position in order to prevent possible aspiration. The interdental gap can be widened with various retractors. The soft palate can often be elevated with a malleable self-retainer. Alternatively, two Red Robin catheters can be fed through nares and brought out from the mouth. The ends on each side is tensioned superolaterally and secured into the drapes. A retraction of the soft palate superiorly with a suture and transnasal rubber catheter is also an option. Although surgical loupes with overhead illumination can be used in these cases, an operating microscope provides a clearer image and allows for easier assistant participation.

11.1.2 Technique

Incision: The entrance to the oral cavity between the upper and lower incisors must be at least 2.5–3.0 cm in order to have adequate loupe or microscope visualization and introduce instruments (Fig. 11.2). A midline incision is made into the posterior pharynx extending from the rostral clivus to the C2–C3 interspace, exposing the prevertebral fascia and longus colli muscles. These tissues are dissected laterally revealing the clivus, the anterior arch of the atlas and the odontoid peg (Fig. 11.3a). The incision is made full thickness to bone through the mucosa and pharyngeal musculature. If additional superior exposure is required, the soft palate may be incised in the midline starting on one side of the

Fig. 11.2 The transoral approach to the axis

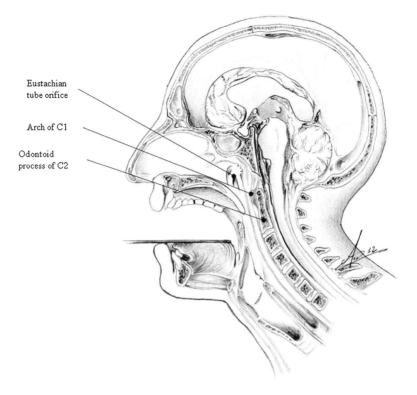

Eustachian tube orifice

Arch of C1

Odontoid process of C2

base of the uvula and laterally retracted. Subperiosteal dissection of the anterior longitudinal ligament is done with electrocautery and should be carried out from the midline. Lateral elevation on the atlas should be restricted to 1.5 cm from the midline (the width of the exposure is maintained at approximately 3 cm), as the vertebral arteries, internal carotid arteries, and hypoglossal nerves are at risk with more aggressive lateral exposure (Fig. 11.3b). The internal carotid artery can be quite close to the midline, as suggested by Currier et al. [8], who found it more than 7.5 mm medial to the foramen transversarium in 6 % of their subjects [8]. The hypoglossal nerve lies approximately 2–3 mm lateral to the middle of the anterior aspect of the lateral mass of the atlas [9]. If access to the odontoid is desired, the central 1–1.5 cm of the atlas may be resected to expose the upper portion of the axis. The anterior arch of the atlas is drilled out, and the inferior clivus is remove. The dural circular sinus (basilar plexus) has to be carefully dissected off the inferior border of the clivus to prevent hemorrhage and/or dural injury and a subsequent cerebrospinal fluid leak. The anterior portion of the atlas should be removed, attempt to preserve the transverse ligament, if possible. The transverse ligament prevents lateral displacement of the atlas lateral masses, which can lead to craniocervical instability. If it cannot be preserved, a posterior occipitocervical arthrodesis may be necessary.

11.1.3 Extensions

It may be combined with palatal or mandibular splitting procedures for additional rostral and caudal exposure [10].

11.2 Lateral Approach

In 1966, Whiteside's and Kelly introduced the lateral approach to the upper cervical spine as an alternative to the anterior transmucosal and anterolateral retropharyngeal approaches [5].

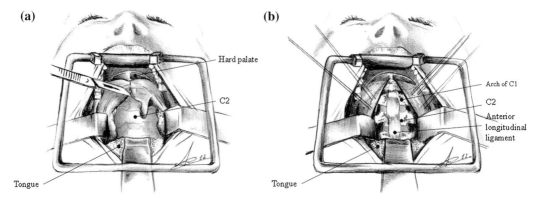

Fig. 11.3 The transoral approach to the axis

This approach was based on the one used by Henry to expose the vertebral artery between the atlas and axis [11]. Henry's technique emphasized the dorsal reflection of the sternocleidomastoid muscle after its division at the mastoid process, thereby allowing direct lateral exposure of the vertebral artery via blunt dissection.

Several modifications of the lateral approach to the upper cervical spine have been published [12–22] focused in particular indications. Babu [21] and Salas [22] were the first to introduce the term "extreme lateral transfacetal approach". Their approach also included hemilaminectomy of the atlas and axis, and it is mainly used for non-osseous lesions arising in the canal.

The lateral approach as it was introduced by Barbour, popularized by DuToit and Simmons and modified by the team of "La Pitie-Salpetriere" (11–16) is nowadays used. This technique is used in cases where there is no possible to perform a posterior atlantoaxial arthrodesis like in the case of a fracture of the posterior arch of the Atlas, of a Jefferson fracture associated to a fracture of the odontoid process, in case of a failed posterior arthrodesis, in case of previous atlantoaxial laminectomy or in the presence of instability due to congenital malformations (agenesis or hypoplasty of the posterior arch of the Atlas) and in case of pseudarthosis of an odontoid fracture.

The patient is placed in a supine position while a pillow is placed under the shoulder at the operative side and the head is turned slightly to the opposite side. The arthrodesis is done bilaterally - as the unilateral atlantoaxial fixation is not a stable one—under x-ray control. The ear is pushed out of the operative field by means of a suture.

The incision of about 6 cm starts at the base of the mastoid and curved along the anterior border of the sternomastoid muscle which is identified as well as the greater auricular nerve and external jugular vein. After detachment of the origin of the anterior belly of the sternomastoid and retracting posteriorly the muscle we cut the prevertable fascia revealing deep to it the transverse process of the atlas. The muscles attached to the transverse (anterior oblique and angular) are sectioned. A retractor is placed in order to keep the neurovascular bundle anteriorly giving easy access to the lateral mass of the Atlas and the atlantoaxial joint. By mobilization of the head we can reduce now the atlantoaxial joint and insert a 26 mm long navicular lag screw. The inter-transverse muscles are respected to protect the vertebral artery in the transverse canal. The anterior side of the transverse apophysis of there axis is exposed to point out the atlantoaxial joints and the lateral masses of the atlas and axis. The longus colli muscles is detached from the anterior body of the atlas and axis, and displaced forward. It is possible to reach the anterior tubercle of the atlas in the retropharyngeal space. With a bilateral approach the two surgeons can meet at this level. The atlantoaxial joint can be exposed very well using a Homann lever fixed to the odontoid base. If a larger approach on the lateral masses of the atlas and axis is necessary, it must open the transverse canal removing the external anterior part. The vertebral artery can be mobilized or tied.

The direction of the screw is 25° below to the horizontal in the coronal plane and slightly posterior. Before fixing the screw the joint is prepared by a curatte and filled with bone chips. The wound is closed after reinsertion of the sternomastoid and application of a suction drain. The same procedure is done to the opposite side.

The modification proposed by Roy-Camille et al. [16, 17] concern the approach not through the anterior border of the sternocleidomastoid muscle, but through its two heads. In this approach the potential for complications is low.

Advantage:
- Less risk of infection, being extraoral.

Disadvantages:
- Damage of the vertebral artery with bleeding difficult to control.
- Not approachable the contralateral vertebral artery.
- The anterior decompression of the spinal cord is more difficult due to narrow and deep access.
- More difficult reconstruction to insert long strut grafts in patients in whom the lesion spans several vertebral bodies.

11.3 Antero-Lateral Approach

11.3.1 Above the Hyoid Bone

This approach guarantees a good exposure of the antero-lateral part of the body of the atlas and axis.

This is the higher part of the classic anterior approach to the cervical spine. Anterior retropharyngeal approach was described by McAfee [23]. It is excellent for anterior debridement of the upper cervical spine. It is relatively easy to extend this distally, through a more classic Smith-Robertson approach, to access the lower cervical spine, if necessary. It is entirely extramucosal and has fewer complications as far as

wound infection and neurological deficit are concerned.

11.3.1.1 Preoperative Planning

Particular attention should be focused on any compromise of swallowing or respiratory function. In the revision setting, it may be necessary to have the patient undergo vocal cord evaluation. A preoperative tracheotomy may be warranted for avoiding airway problems, and an otolaryngologist can assist with this determination. In this approach a preoperative visualization of the vertebral arteries is necessary if radiographic images show involvement of the foramen transversarium at the second cervical level, or tumour is displacing the vertebral arteries. This evaluation is also used to localize the major feeding vessels of the tumour [23]. This approach is difficult because in this side there are many vascular and nervous structures. The surgeon must be familiar with the fascial planes that are traversed by this approach: (1) the superficial fascia containing the platysma; (2) the superficial layer of the deep fascia surrounding the sternocleidomastoid muscle; (3) the middle layer of the deep fascia that enclosed the omohyoid, sternohyoid, sternothyroid and thyrohyoid muscles and the visceral fascia enclosing the trachea, esophagus, and recurrent nerve; (4) the deep layer of the deep cervical fascia which is divided into the alar fascia connecting the two carotid sheaths and fused in the midline to the cervical fascia and the prevertebral fascia covering the longus colli and scalene muscle (Fig. 11.4).

11.3.1.2 Position

The procedure is performed with the patient positioned supine with the head in mild extension and rotated 30–45° away from the side of the approach. The approach can be made either from the left or the right side, since the high extra pharyngeal approach is sufficiently superior to the right recurrent laryngeal nerve. A cranial traction should be strongly considered. If postoperative halo-vest immobilization is

Fig. 11.4 Anterior retropharyngeal approach to upper cervical spine: *cross section drawing. m* muscle

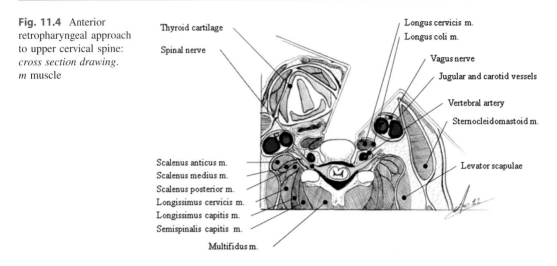

planned, the use of a halo ring can be substituted for Gardner-Wells tongs. Before traction is applied, baseline evoked potentials from neuromonitoring should be obtained (if used). The patient should be awake for fiberoptic Nasotracheal intubation, so neurologic assessment can be performed following the intubation and positioning. Oral placement of tubes or devices should be avoided, as they may inferiorly displace the mandible and compromise maximum exposure of the upper-most aspects of the cervical spine. Finally, place the patient in a slight reverse-Trendelenburg position to aid in visualization and improve venous drainage. The ipsilateral earlobe should be prepped and then sutured to the cheek anteriorly. Otherwise, it will be an obstruction during the exposure.

11.3.1.3 Technique

Although this approach can be carried out medial (anterior approach) or lateral (anterolateral approach) to the carotid sheath, the anterior retropharyngeal approach is preferred [23]. By accessing the retropharyngeal space medial to the carotid sheath, one avoids the risk of injuring the carotid vessels or cranial nerves at the skull base, but there is a higher risk of injury to the superior laryngeal or glossopharyngeal nerves than when approached lateral to the carotid sheath. Some authors suggest a left-side approach to decrease the risk of injury to the

recurrent laryngeal nerve. They support that the left nerve is less vulnerable to injury than the right nerve because it is vertical and ascends to the tracheoesophageal groove. However, the axis is sufficiently superior to the right recurrent laryngeal nerve. The recurrent laryngeal nerve can not be damaged if the approach does not have to be extended below the level of the fifth cervical vertebra. Therefore, a right-sided exposure in the upper cervical spine is convenient for a right-handed surgeon. Additionally, the anterior approach allows access to both vertebral arteries, while exposing lateral to the carotid sheath compromises access to the contralateral vertebral artery. Finally, anterior decompression and reconstructive measures may be more easily performed when visualizing the spine from the anterior approach than the anterolateral approach.

The submandibular incision, also known as the modified Schoebringer incision, is used for this approach. The submandibular incision for the anterior approach begins at the midline just under the mandible, at level of the hyoid bone, arched 2 cm below the body of the mandible, and curved superiorly toward the mastoid tip (Fig. 11.5). Sometimes, a T-shaped incision is performed with a transverse skin incision in the submandibular region with a vertical extension as long as required to provide adequate exposure is made. The vertical limb extends inferiorly only as far as it is needed, depending on the

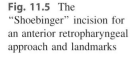

Fig. 11.5 The "Shoebinger" incision for an anterior retropharyngeal approach and landmarks

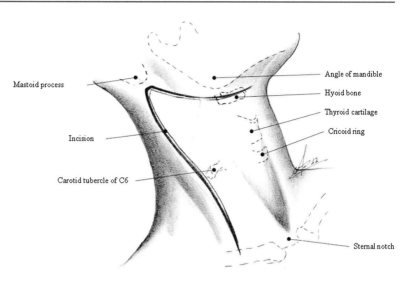

Mastoid process

Incision

Carotid tubercle of C6

Angle of mandible

Hyoid bone

Thyroid cartilage

Cricoid ring

Sternal notch

amount of cervical spine that must be exposed. Considering the looseness of skin in this location, a modified less invasive curving incision is suggested in an effort to make the caudal extension easier. The skin incision begins two fingerbreadths in front of the angle of mandible, proceeds one fingerbreadth below the mandible and curves downward across the submandibular triangle and carotid triangle. The caudal exposure can be extended easily if needed. Downward extension of the incision connects with the routing anterior cervical approach which offers caudal exposure for lower cervical vertebral bodies. Riley [6] suggested a modified incision that begun just to the left of the midline in the submandibular area in a skin crease, carried posterior to the angle of the mandible, then directed in a gentle curve lateral to the posterior border of the sternomastoid muscle to the level of the fifth cervical segment, curved anteriorly and inferiorly crossing the clavicle and ending in the suprasternal space. The large flap with skin, subcutaneous fascia, platysma muscle is reflected medially to expose the sternomastoid muscle, the strap muscle, the pharynx, the thyroid gland, the edge of mandible and the submaxillary fossa (Fig. 11.6). The sternomastoid muscle and the carotid sheath are retracted laterally and the esophagus, the trachea, the thyroid gland medially. The anterior surface of the mid and lower cervical spine is visualized. The skin and superficial fascia are incised in line with the incision. The platysma muscle and the superficial fascia are dissected and retracted exposing the inferior edge of the submandibular gland. Then the submandibular gland is elevated and the fascial capsule is opened and dissected horizontally (Fig. 11.7). The facial artery and vein are identified and dissected free in the field of dissection posterior and lateral to the gland. Before proceeding more deeply, a nerve stimulator can be used to find the mandibular branch of the facial nerve that should be preserved due to its innervation of the orbicularis oris muscle. The marginal mandibular branch of the seventh cranial nerve is identified by ligating and retracting the retromandibular vein. The common facial vein is continuous with the retromandibular vein and the branches of the marginal mandibular nerve usually cross the vein superficially and superiorly. By ligating the retromandibular vein superiorly as it joins the internal jugular vein and keeping the dissection deep and inferior to the vein as the exposure is extended superiorly to the mandible, the superficial branches of the facial nerve are protected. The facial vein, which runs superficial to the parotid gland, can be found and ligated just inferior to the submandibular gland. It typically courses superficial to the gland and is oriented cephalocaudally. By leaving the ligature on the superior stump of the vein, it can be

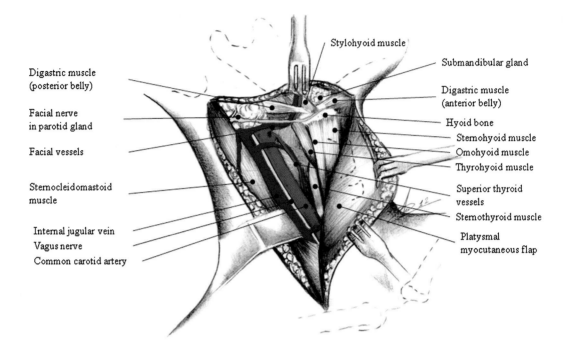

Fig. 11.6 Superficial dissection for the anterior retropharyngeal approach

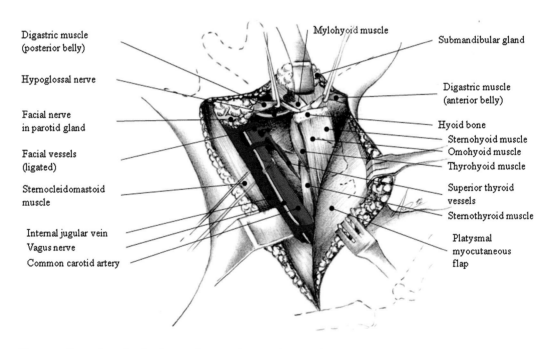

Fig. 11.7 Deep dissection for the anterior retropharyngeal approach

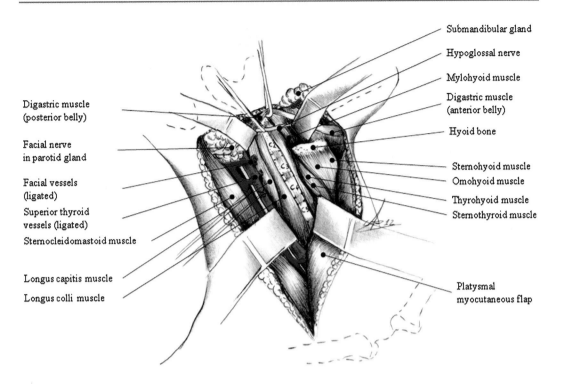

Digastric muscle
(posterior belly)

Facial nerve
in parotid gland

Facial vessels
(ligated)

Superior thyroid
vessels (ligated)

Sternocleidomastoid muscle

Longus capitis muscle

Longus colli muscle

Submandibular gland

Hypoglossal nerve

Mylohyoid muscle

Digastric muscle
(anterior belly)

Hyoid bone

Sternohyoid muscle

Omohyoid muscle

Thyrohyoid muscle

Sternothyroid muscle

Platysmal
myocutaneous flap

Fig. 11.8 Further deep dissection for the anterior retropharyngeal approach

used to retract the superficial fascia of the sub-mandibular gland and protect the marginal branch of the mandibular nerve as it courses within the fascia. The submandibular salivary gland was mobilized superiorly (or it can be resected in short necks) to access the prevertebral area from below the mandible, exposing the intersection of digastric and stylohyoid muscles. These muscles are divided at their confluence near the hyoid bone and reflected proximally. Occasionally, the submandibular gland must be resected to allow adequate exposure; however, its corresponding salivary duct must then be ligated to prevent fistula formation. Next, the superior thyroid, lingual, and facial arteries and associated veins are ligated and divided (Fig. 11.8). It is helpful to proceed from inferior to superior during this process, using the hyoid bone as a marker for localizing each artery. The superior thyroid artery is just below the hyoid bone, while the lingual and facial arteries are at and just above it, respectively. The superior laryngeal nerve often travels close to the superior thyroid artery, and injury to it must be

avoided. The anterior border of the sternocleidomastoid muscle is mobilized by longitudinally dividing the superficial layer of the deep cervical fascia. This allows localization of the carotid sheath and the content of the carotid sheath is protected. The jugular-digastric lymph nodes from the submandibular and carotid triangle can be resected and a frozen biopsy is possible. Dissection of the stylohyoid and the posterior belly of the digastric muscle allowed medial mobilization of the hyoid bone and hypopharynx so to prevent exposure of the esophagus, hypopharynx and nasopharynx and traction on the facial nerve that could be injured by superior retraction on the stylohyoid muscle. The muscle bellies are then retracted upward to reveal the external and internal carotids and the hypoglossal trunk. The hypoglossal nerve is completely mobilized from the base of the skull to the anterior border of the hypoglossal muscle. It is gently identified and retracted superiorly. The fascia between the hyoid bone and carotid sheath is incised and the carotid sheath is then retracted laterally. The dissection extends to the

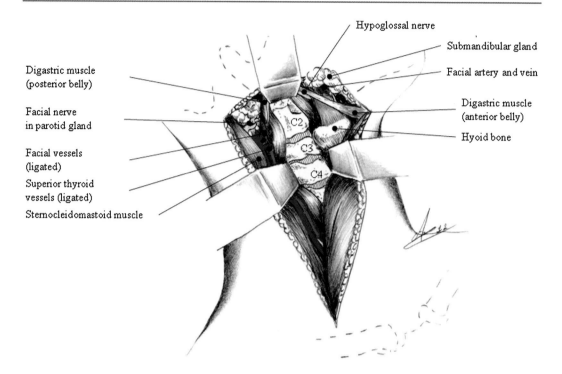

Digastric muscle (posterior belly)

Facial nerve in parotid gland

Facial vessels (ligated)

Superior thyroid vessels (ligated)

Sternocleidomastoid muscle

Hypoglossal nerve

Submandibular gland

Facial artery and vein

Digastric muscle (anterior belly)

Hyoid bone

C2

C3

C4

Fig. 11.9 View of the atlantoaxial region through the anterior retropharyngeal approach

retropharyngeal space between the carotid sheath laterally and the larynx and pharynx medially. The exposure is increased by ligating branches of the carotid artery and internal jugular vein which prevent retraction of the carotid sheath laterally. Beginning inferiorly and progressing superiorly, ligating the following branches of these vessels helps mobilize the carotid sheath laterally: (1) superior thyroid artery and vein, (2) lingual artery and vein, (3) ascending pharyngeal artery and vein, (4) facial artery and vein. The superior laryngeal nerve which courses deeply and parallel to the superior thyroid artery in the paratracheal fascia is identified and mobilized from its origin near the nodose ganglion to its entrance into the larynx. After the dissection medial to the carotid bundle was completed, the hypoglossal nerve is found medial to the tendon of the digastric muscle, more superior than the superior laryngeal nerve; both should be protected by careful dissection and mobilization. Once the hypoglossal nerve is dissected out from its exiting site at the skull base to its insertion near the tongue, it can be

retracted rostrally and the cervical vertebral bodies were thus exposed from the atlas to C3 (Fig. 11.9). After an adequate retraction of the carotid sheath laterally, the retropharyngeal space is opened and the alar fascia, prevertebral fascial layers are divide longitudinally away from the longus colli muscles with a peanut or Kittner dissector. Although medial retraction of the pharynx is helpful, excessive force can cause iatrogenic injury to the laryngeal and pharyngeal branches of the vagus nerve. Use blunt finger dissection to separate the carotid sheath from the medial pharynx and larynx, and the retropharyngeal space can then be safely entered. The longus colli muscles are exposed and they are then divided longitudinally in the midline. The longus colli muscles insert on the anterior arch of the atlas bilaterally, so they can help define the midline of the atlas if adequately exposed. The head has to be maintained in a neutral position and the midline has to be accurately identified by noting the attachment of the left and right longus colli muscles as they converge toward the anterior tubercle of the atlas. The amount of rotation of the head away from the midline is gauged by palpating the mental protuberance of the mandible. Visualization of the uncovertebral joints between these vertebrae helps to confirm the orientation of the midline. This orientation must be maintained as the longus colli muscles are detached from the anterior surface of the atlas and axis. The muscles are removed subperiosteally from the anterior arch of the atlas and the body of the axis and then elevated in a lateral and cephalad direction. When starting the midline incision, avoid extending beyond the cephalad margin of the atlas, which could violate the anterior occipito atlantal membrane. The anterior longitudinal ligament underlying the longus colli should be reflected within these flaps. The decompression may be carried far enough laterally as to decompress the spinal cord but not so far laterally as to endanger the vertebral arteries. Limit lateral elevation of these flaps on the atlas to 1.5 cm from midline, as the vertebral arteries can be in significant danger beyond this distance. The posterior longitudinal ligament may be removed as necessary for visualization of the cord. If decompression is planned, it should generally be performed in a cephalad-to-caudal direction. This reduces difficulty with visualization, as bleeding tends to run in a caudal direction. The posterior longitudinal ligament and uncovertebral joints help identify the posterior and lateral safety margins of the decompression. The anterior decompression is usually initiated by removing the intervertebral disc between the axis and C3 or the first normal disc at the caudal edge of the lesion. If reconstruction is to be performed, the head should be carefully repositioned to neutral alignment prior to graft placement and fixation. The wound is closed after copious irrigation in reverse order through which the approach was made over suction drains after repairing the digastric tendon, the platysma and superficial fascia. After treatment, the patient is maintained in skeletal traction with the head of the bed elevated 30° to reduce hypopharyngeal edema. Intubation is continued from 12 to 72 h after surgery to prevent possible airway obstruction which might be caused by

edema in the pharynx and retropharyngeal space. Initial parenteral nutrition is administrated for the first two postoperative days and then nasogastric feeding or liquid diet is begun. A hard cervical collar or Philadelphia type collar is maintained related to the surgical reconstruction or stabilization.

Advantages:
- Greater degree of bilateral exposure than the transoral and lateral approach (type a),
- Less risk of infection,
- Simultaneous instrumentations during the primary surgical procedure,
- Provides a safer environment for intradural procedure and management of a cerebral spinal fluid leak,
- Does not require a tracheostomy and thus its complications are avoided,
- Can also provide exposure of the retropharyngeal midline foramen magnum and the lower clivus.

Risks:
- Risk of injury to the marginal mandibular branch, hypoglossal and superior laryngeal nerves, with a transient dysphagia and dysphonia often for few days but sometimes for several months. Neuropraxia is a not uncommon complication of this approach.
- Airway obstruction secondary to edema or bone grafting into the posterior pharynx is the most immediate threat. Tracheostomy intubation may be considered if prolonged intubation is thought to be necessary.

11.3.2 Below the Hyoid Bone

This approach provides with a wide exposure of the distal cervical spine.

This approach is used to reach the upper cervical spine avoiding many vascular and nervous structures that are met in the previous approach. The same tract is used for the distal cervical spine. A vertical incision along 5 cm in front of the sternomastoid muscle from the mid level of the neck to the hyoid bone is performed. The first contact with the spine is a C4 level. Usually, the superior thyroid artery is ligated.

The superior laryngeal nerve, medially to the external carotid artery and down to the lingual artery, can be moved out and down. With a gentle dissection of the aero-digestive axis and with a soft and medial traction of the pharyngeal muscles from the bottom upwards, the spine is exposed. The upper cervical spine is cleared from the midline subperiosteally so to arrive from the C2–C3 junction to the odontoid base that is located in the axis of the instruments and it is seen directly from the bottom upwards. It is possible to go up the spine to the edge of the body of the axis anterior tubercle of which it is palpable with the fingers. Some right and long spatula can enlarge the wound but this approach remains narrow and deep.

11.4 Posterior Approach

The midline posterior approach is the most commonly used approach to the cervical spine, allowing quick and safe access to the posterior elements of the entire cervical spine.

11.4.1 Preoperative Planning

- Flexion and extension views to assess for segmental instability prior to decompression or fusion.
- CT scan to provide more accurate detail of the bony anatomy.
- Patient's body habitus and posterior neck skin condition to adjustments to the planned approach.

11.4.2 Position

Neuromonitoring is encouraged for most procedures in this region of the spine. Once baseline monitoring has been established, intubation can proceed. The patient is then placed in the prone position on an operating table, with the head into a few degrees of flexion to open the interspinous spaces. For procedures in the posterior cervical spine, it is helpful to have the arms located at the sides during surgery. A special head brace or a padded ring may be used to control position of the head during surgery. The relationship of the occiput to the upper cervical spine should be optimized to prevent postoperative swallowing dysfunction, which may result from fusing the occipital cervical area in a non-physiologic position. Positioning should be performed with the patient under light sedation to allow a wake-up test following positioning, to assure maintenance of neurologic integrity. Reverse-Trendelenburg position of the operating table facilitates visualization of the occipitocervical junction, and may also reduce venous congestion and bleeding during surgery.

11.4.3 Technique

Incision: from external occipital tubercle for 6–8 cm. to the bottom in the midline (Fig. 11.10). An epinephrine solution, with or without local anesthetic, can be injected in the subdermal layer along the line of the planned midline incision to decrease bleeding from the skin edges. Use the electrocautery to dissect through the subcutaneous fat in the midline. It is sometimes helpful to gently clear subcutaneous fat off of the midline nuchal fascia, to aid in identifying the proper planes during closure. Once the nuchal fascia is identified, finger palpation may be utilized to assure that the incision is in the midline (Fig. 11.11). The spinous process of the axis should be readily apparent as the most prominent upper cervical vertebra at this point. Use electrocautery to divide the nuchal fascia in the midline and elevate the flaps slightly in both lateral directions from the underlying paraspinal musculature. This will expose an avascular plane lateral to the interspinalis cervicis muscles on either side of the spinous process and will aid in preservation of the interspinous ligaments. Take care to prevent violation of the C2–C3 interspinous ligament, unless this segment is planned for inclusion in decompression or fusion. Once the nuchal fascia has been divided, palpate the spinous processes

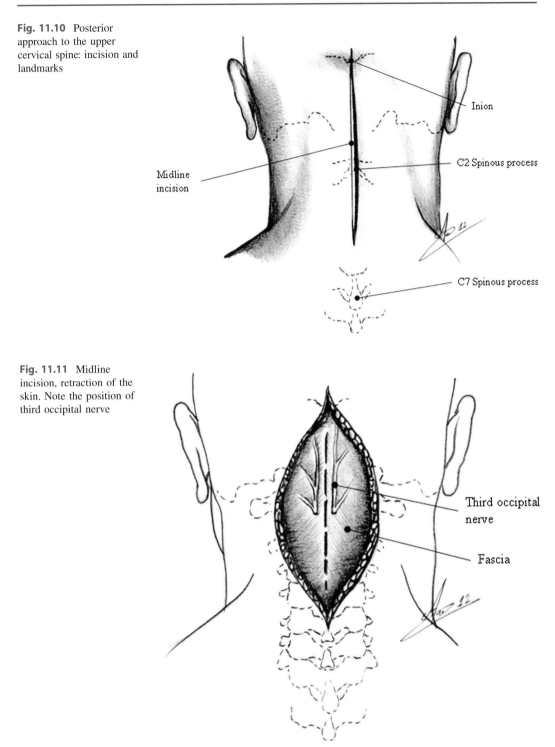

Fig. 11.10 Posterior approach to the upper cervical spine: incision and landmarks

Inion

Midline incision

C2 Spinous process

C7 Spinous process

Fig. 11.11 Midline incision, retraction of the skin. Note the position of third occipital nerve

Third occipital nerve

Fascia

for orientation. The most prominent spinous process rostrally is that of the axis and the most distal bifid spinous process is usually C6. An intraoperative radiograph is essential to confirm the level because anatomic variations are common. Although access to the deeper structures

Fig. 11.12 Exposure of
the lamina and facet joints
of the cervical vertebrae

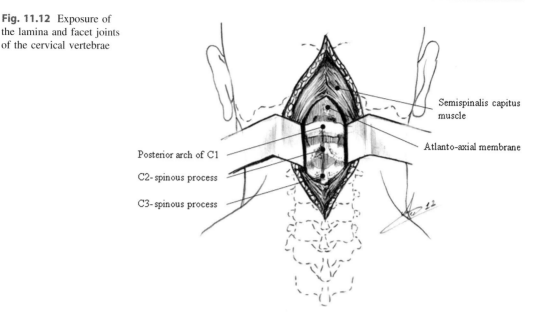

Semispinalis capitus
muscle

Atlanto-axial membrane

Posterior arch of C1

C2-spinous process

C3-spinous process

through this avascular plane is not critical, the reduction in bleeding afforded by this technique facilitates hemostasis and visualization during surgery. The greater occipital nerve courses through the fascia and can be injured if the exposure strayed from the midline or at the end of surgery if fascial sutures are placed too far laterally. Gently palpate the bony anatomy once again and note the depth of the posterior arch of C1 for orientation. Electrocautery can be used to incise down to bone on the occiput, as well as to perform a subperiosteal elevation from the laminae of the axis. Muscles released from the axis include the rectus capitis major and the obliquus capitis inferior, but muscles directed caudally from the spinous process of the axis (semispinalis cervicis) should be preserved unless access to the caudal aspect of the spinous process of the axis is critical. Unless the C2–C3 segment must be fused, the C2–C3 articular capsules should be preserved. This capsular layer is often wispy and difficult to recognize, but it plays an important role in posterior stability. If the semispinalis cervicis must be released, elevate the insertion of the muscle with a thin piece of bone using an osteotome. The muscle attachment can then be repaired anatomically and securely at the end of

the case. Sharp dissection with a scalpel can now be carried down to the posterior arch of the atlas in the midline. This maneuver should only be performed if adequate preoperative computed tomography or intraoperative palpation confirms an intact posterior ring. Use a Cobb elevator, which can remove the muscles from the bone without damaging them unduly. Extreme caution should be employed when elevating laterally off of the arch of the atlas, limiting the dissection on the cephalad aspect of the atlas to 0.8 cm from the midline, as the vertebral arteries can be easily injured beyond this point. Rarely, the posterior ring of the atlas can be nonconfluent or absent. Continue gentle blunt dissection to lift paraspinal musculature away from base of the occiput and off of the atlantoaxial junction superficial to the level of the lamina (Fig. 11.12). Carry the dissection as far laterally as necessary to reveal the lamina, the facet joints, and the beginnings of the transverse processes. If necessary, the atlantoaxial membrane may be carefully elevated from the arch of the atlas and lamina of the axis with a curette to expose the dura. The venous plexus surrounding the C2 nerve roots and ganglions become visible as the atlantoaxial articulation is approached.

11.4.4 Extensions

The exposure can be enlarged starting the incision at the external occipital protuberance and extends to the spinous process of C7. Sharp dissection is made to have a subperiosteal exposure of the squamous-occipital bone and the bony elements of the upper cervical spine as necessary. The dissection of the small rotator muscles from the occipital squama and the region of foramen magnum must be performed with a sharp knife. In some cases the foramen magnum can only be reached after the laminectomy of the atlas is accomplished. Otherwise, the posterior fossa craniectomy and the upper cervical laminectomy can be necessary and performed with a high-speed drill. Reconstitution of the dura, sometimes with a dural graft, is essential.

References

1. Lahey FH, Warren KW (1954) Esophageal diverticula. Surg Gynec Obstet 98:1–28
2. Southwick WO, Robinson RA (1957) Surgical approaches to the vertebral bodies in the cervical and lumbar regions. J Bone Joint Surg 39-A:631–644
3. Robinson RA (1959) Fusion of the cervical spine. J Bone Joint Surg 41-A:1–6
4. Fang HS, Ong GB (1962) Direct anterior approach to the upper cervical spine. J Bone Joint Surg 44-A:1588–1604
5. Whitesides TE, Kelly RP (1966) Lateral approach to the upper cervical spine for anterior fusion. Southern Med J 59:879–883
6. Riley LH (1973) Surgical approaches to the anterior cervical spine. Clin Orthop 91:16
7. Hall JE, Denis F, Murray J (1977) Exposure of the upper cervical spine for spinal decompression by a mandible and tongue-splitting approach. J Bone Joint Surg 59A:121–123
8. Currier B, Yaszemski M (2004) The use of C1 lateral mass fixation in the cervical spine. Curr Opin Orthop 15(3):184–191
9. Ebraheim NA, Misson JR, Xu R et al (2000) The optimal transarticular C1–2 screw length and the location of the hypoglossal nerve. Surg Neurol 53(3):208–210
10. Youssef AS, Sloan AE (2010) Extended transoral approaches: surgical technique and analysis. Neurosurgery 66(3 Suppl):126–34
11. Henry AK (1966) Extensile exposure. Churchill livingstone, Edinburgh, pp 58–72
12. Barbour JR (1971) Screw fixation and fractures of the odontoid process. S Aust Chir Vol 5:20–24
13. Du Toit G (1976) Lateral atlanto-axial arthrodesis. A screw fixation technique. S Afr J Surg 14:9–12
14. Smmons HE, Dutoit G (1978) Lateral atlantoaxial arthrodesis. Orth Clin North Am 9:1101–1114
15. Feron JM (1981) Abord chirurgical lateral des massifs articulaires de l' atlas et de l' axis: technique et indications. These Medecine, Paris
16. Roy-Camille R, Bouchet T, Saillant G, Feron JM (1986) Technique de l' abord lateral de C1–C2. In: Rachis cervical superieur. Cinquiemes journees de la Pitie. Masson, Paris
17. Roy-Camille R, Mazel CHR (1992) Voie d'abord. In: Atlas de chirurgie orthopedique (tome 1er) generalites, rahis. Masson, Paris pp 297–356
18. Al-Mefty O, Borba LAB, Aoki N, Angtuaco E, Pait TG (1996) The transcondylar approach to extradural nonneoplastic lesions of the craniovertebral junction. J Neurosurg 84:1–6
19. George B (1998) Exposure of the upper cervical vertebral artery. In: Dickman CA, Spetzler RF, Sonntag VKH (eds) Surgery of the craniovertebral junction. Thieme, New York, pp 545–567
20. Shucart WA, Kleriga E (1980) Lateral approach to the upper cervical spine. Neurosurgery 6:278–281
21. Babu RP, Sekhar LN, Wright DC (1994) Extreme lateral transcondylar approach: technical improvements and lessons learned. J Neurosurg 81(1):49–59
22. Salas E, Sekhar LN, Ziyal IM, Caputy AJ, Wright DC (1999) Variations of the extreme-lateral craniocervical approach: anatomical study and clinical analysis of 69 patients. J Neurosurg 90(2 Suppl):206–19
23. McAfee PC, Bohlman HH, Riley LH et al (1987) The anterior retropharyngeal approach to the upper part of the cervical spine. J Bone Joint Surg 69-A:1371–1383

Transmandible Approach

12

Carlo Logroscino, Luca Proietti, Giovanni Almadori
and Gaetano Paludetti

The anterior approach to the upper cervical spine, often mandatory for tumor resection, represents a challenging procedure associated with risks and uncertainties regarding the selection of the appropriate surgical plan. Transoral and extraoral approaches are available, and the literature offers a variety of different descriptions of surgical exposures and modifications to improve the visualization of a lesion, create more favorable conditions for the reconstruction and reduce the complication rate.

Transoral surgery is applicable to a limited number of cases involving disorders in the upper *cervical spine* (C1–C2). The reasons are the need for tracheostomy, the danger related with the anatomy of the surgical area. A majority of surgeons are unfamiliar with this approach, and the complication rate described in the literature is high. Indeed, there were few possibilities of using this approach whose first application dates back to the pre-Christian Era and the days of Hippocrates.

The transoral approach has been occasionally used for many years. Various reports on this approach appeared from time to time, but these were actually no more than sporadic reports. The first description in detail and case presentation was given by Fang and Ong in Hong Kong [1]. Like most pioneering efforts a considerable number of complications were encountered and had to be resolved during the preliminary work. Yet, it must be recognized that these surgeons initiated prospects on a procedure which until that time had been considered beset with uncertainties. *Transoral surgery* came to be accepted as the natural anterior approach to the upper cervical spine. The reasons for the serious complications reported in the first operations are not difficult to identify. Infection occurred partly as a consequence of the particular site involved (oral cavity) and partly because of the inadequacy of preoperative preparations and postoperative care. Complications involving hemorrhage (vertebral artery) were attributed to the fact that this technique still required improvement and development. Respiratory failure was probably the result of insufficient assistance and diagnostic unexpertise in the delicate postoperative period. It could well be that Fang and Ong's experience was the consequence of the enthusiasm aroused in Hong Kong by the results achieved by Hodgson and Stock [2] which made possible the anterior approach to the thoracolumbar spine for the treatment of Pott's disease.

C. Logroscino (✉) · L. Proietti
Orthopaedic Department, Catholic University
Rome, Largo Francesco Vito, 8, Rome, 00168, Italy
e-mail: studio@carlologroscino.it

L. Proietti
e-mail: proiettil@yahoo.it

G. Almadori · G. Paludetti
Otorhinolaryngology Department, Catholic
University Rome, Largo Francesco Vito, 8, Rome,
00168, Italy
e-mail: giovannialmadori@rm.unicatt.it

G. Paludetti
e-mail: gaetanopaludetti@rm.unicatt.it

D. S. Korres (ed.), *The Axis Vertebra*,
DOI: 10.1007/978-88-470-5232-1_12, © Springer-Verlag Italia 2013

Nevertheless, transoral surgery has several advantages [3]; it is extremely useful if occipitocervical rigidity is present due to previous fusion, and it allows for direct exposure of the midline without rotation of the head. On the other hand, rotation of the head is essential using an extraoral approach and this may result in a more difficult open reduction and internal fixation. Transoral surgery requires limited dissection and is ideal for urgent spinal cord decompression. Morbidity has decreased significantly over time. We feel that this is an excellent approach allowing the most direct exposure to the front of the upper cervical spine and the best view on both sides of the area (left and right). A significant disadvantage is the limited surgical exposure. This approach, especially in tumors, offers a very small surgical field. It must be stressed, however, that natural obstacles, such as the tongue and mandible, exist that prevent exposure proximally and distally. Correct tumor resection can be difficult to perform; small, fine, precise movements are needed due to space restrictions. Experience and adequate technical equipment are necessary to overcome these limitations. Another limitation involves the impossibility of checking on lesions distal to C2 under normal conditions.

A step forward appeared to be necessary for major resections of pathological tissues and subsequent reconstructions. One of the first attempts in this direction was presented by Schmelzle and Harms [4–6] who described the *extended transoral approach* allowing for improved reconstructive procedures. The surgical technique of extended transoral approach provides the soft palate split and incision of the posterior pharynx mucosa creating a lateral-based door-like flap. Some authors showed that extension of transoral approach in cranial or caudal direction provides to enlarge the surgical field making it more superficial [7].

Crockard introduced a demanding technique called "open door maxillotomy" to allow an approach to the lower clivus using midline maxillary splitting in addition to Le Fort type maxillotomy [8]. Many surgical modifications have been developed in order to enhance the

transoral exposure in the sagittal plane including *mandibulotomy* (division of the mandible), *mandibuloglossotomy* (division of the mandible and tongue) and palatotomy (division of the hard palate). Mandibuloglossotomy allows to reduce the operative distance and increase the sagittal exposure from the upper third of the clivus to the C4–C5 interspace. Going back to the first reports, a description of a mandible and tongue-splitting approach for surgery to the pharynx and the base of the tongue was given by Kocher in the early years of the past century. Hall, Denis and Murray used this approach for treating a postsurgical kyphosis secondary to a huge posterior craniocervical decompression, responsible for a progressive quadriparesis. The surgical approach allowed for bone grafting from *axis* to C5. The fusion was assisted by halo cast, and the final outcome was successfully reached. This was probably the first utilization of a direct *transmandibular* approach to a spinal deformity reported by a major orthopedic journal [9].

The transmandibular approach, which extends the surgical exposure, is anatomically invasive. The face is involved and requires a team approach. However, with respect to the transoral approach, it enhances the surgical exposure, thus allowing for resection and stabilization on more levels [10]. When the reconstruction is correctly performed, the functional recovery is relatively rapid with limited cosmetic disfigure. The surgical aggressiveness is proportional to the severity of the disease.

Mandibulotomy or mandibular osteotomy is an excellent surgical approach designed to gain access to the oral cavity, oropharynx and parapharyngeal space or anterior skull base for resection of primary tumors otherwise not accessible through the open mouth. Thus, a two-team surgical approach is desirable for safety and completeness of the surgical resection. The otorhinolaryngology (head and neck) surgical team provides the necessary exposure to the spinal surgery team in order to perform the appropriate resection of the tumor and vertebral reconstruction, carefully protecting the anterior surface of the spinal cord. The main indication for this approach is an extradural lesion located from the level of the lower clivus to C4 and from the internal carotid artery to the contralateral internal carotid artery (Fig. 12.1a, b).

12.1 Surgical Procedure

The approach is performed by the otorhinolaryngology surgical team. In all cases, a preliminary tracheostomy under local anesthesia is routinely performed in order to reduce the postoperative morbidity affecting the airway management and to obtain a better access to the tongue and to the mandible without having an endotracheal tube intruding into surgical field.

12.1.1 Mandibulotomy and Glossotomy

The mandibulotomy can be performed in two locations. In the midline, between the central incisors teeth and paramedian between the lateral incisor and the canine tooth. Splitting the mandible in the midline with vertical cut requires extraction of one central incisor tooth in order to avoid the extrusion of both incisor teeth, impairing the cosmetic appearance of the lower dentition. In addition, it also requires the division of the geniohyoid and genioglossus muscles extended to the hyomandibular complex leading, as a consequence, to a delayed functional recovery. Furthermore, using the single straight vertical cut, the immobilization of the mandible is difficult due to significant motion of the two ends of the mandible causing delayed union or malunion with secondary malocclusion. On the other hand, the paramedian mandibulotomy with the medially angled cut avoids the extraction or extrusion of the lateral incisor and canine teeth (more space between the two), preserves the hyomandibular complex and provides a more stable osteotomy for fixation. For these reasons, we prefer a paramedian mandibulotomy.

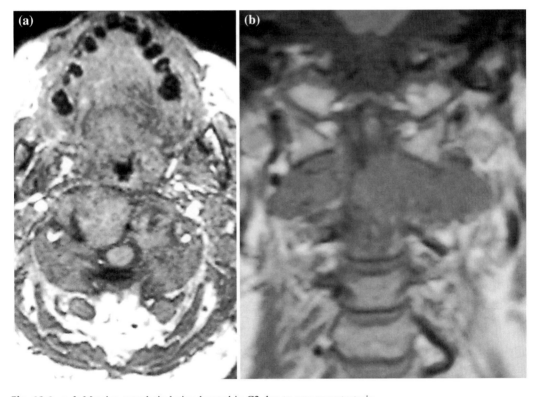

Fig. 12.1 **a, b** Massive osteolytic lesion located in C2 due to cancer metastasis

The patient is positioned supine, the neck is extended, and a vertical midline incision splitting the lower lip and the chin up to the hyoid bone is performed. The skin incision divides the lower lip and the soft tissues of the chin up to the anterior surface of the mandible. Short cheek flaps are elevated on both sides to a distance of 2–3 cm from the midline to expose the lateral cortex and the inferior border of the mandible at the mandibulotomy site. Elevation of the cheek flap should not be extended up to the mental foramen in order to avoid mental nerve injury resulting in loss of sensation of the skin over the chin. The osteotomy site is performed in a vertical plane for 10 mm and then is angled medially, below the level of the roots of adjacent teeth without devitalize them (Fig. 12.2). Before doing the osteotomy and the bony division, appropriate drill holes are performed on the outer cortex and over the lower border of the mandible, aiming to fix the osteotomy by using two titanium *miniplates*, thus assuring an accurate approximation of the two ends of the mandible at the time of closure (Fig. 12.3). After this preliminary and temporary fixation, the miniplates are removed and saved for the final fixation and reconstruction at the end of the operation. The *mandibular osteotomy* is performed exactly as planned using a high-speed power reciprocant saw with

ultra-thin blade. Once the mandibular bone is divided, its two segments are retracted laterally, and the floor of the mouth, frenulum of the tongue and the entire tongue are bisected in the midline from its tip down to the hyoid bone and the median glossoepiglottic fold (Fig. 12.4). Since the blood supply to the tongue arises from the lingual artery on either lateral side, minimal bleeding occurs when the glossotomy is exactly performed in the midline. Similarly, the lingual nerve is always preserved without loss or impairment of the taste sensation. The two halves of the oral cavity and the mandible are then rotated and retracted laterally and inferiorly to expose the oropharynx, the tip and the lingual surface of the epiglottis at the posterior end of the glossotomy and the posterior pharyngeal wall.

12.1.2 Soft Palatal Split

The incision is done after the injection of epinephrine 1:100.000 solution in order to obtain a decongestant effect and carried out through all layers in a safely way. The two halves of the soft palate are retracted laterally and sutured to the self-retaining Dingman retractor which provides the exposure of the posterior pharyngeal wall from the level of the arytenoids to the

Fig. 12.2 The osteotomy site is outlined in a vertical plane for 10 mm and then is angled medially

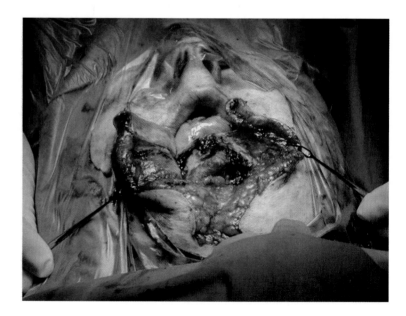

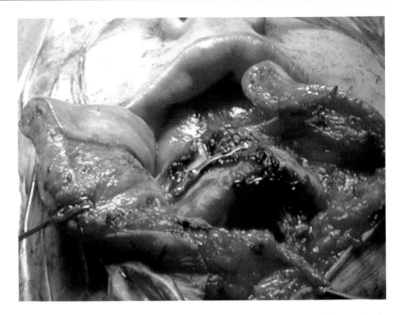

Fig. 12.3 Before doing the osteotomy and the bony division, appropriate drill holes are performed on the outer cortex and over the lower border of the mandible, aiming to fix the osteotomy by using two titanium miniplates, thus assuring an accurate reapproximation of the two ends of the mandible at the time of the closure. After this preliminary and temporary fixation, the miniplates are removed and saved for the final fixation and reconstruction at the end of the operation

nasopharynx. The soft palate can also be divided using a modified midline incision from the lateral base of the uvula to the soft–hard palate in order to preserve its tip and body and to reduce velar incompetence after closure.

12.1.3 Pharyngeal Split

The posterior pharyngeal wall is then injected with decongestant epinephrine solution. A vertical midline incision is carried out dividing the mucosa of the posterior pharyngeal wall, and the incision is deepened through the whole thickness of the pharyngeal musculature to expose the prevertebral fascia. Adequate mobilization of the pharyngeal wall is undertaken over the prevertebral fascia to gain wide exposure of the stretched prevertebral fascia.

12.1.4 Spine Surgical Time

At this point, the visualization of the upper cervical spine from the base of the skull down to C4 is optimal and it is reached without any

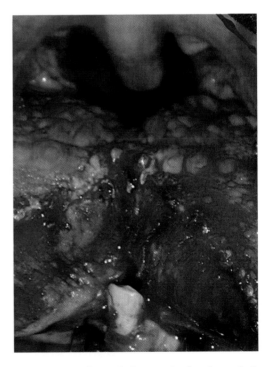

Fig. 12.4 The floor of the mouth, frenulum of the tongue and the entire tongue are bisected in the midline from its tip down to the hyoid bone and the median glossoepiglottic fold

rotation of the head allowing an easy control of both sides of the spine, through a single approach. The self-retaining Crockard pharyngeal retractor may be advantageous. The prevertebral fascia is then incised in the midline and retracted laterally by using anchored Vicryl sutures. It is finally possible to carry out a direct surgical resection of any pathological tissue extended laterally, side to side, and posteriorly toward the dural sac and the spinal cord which can be decompressed under microscopical magnification. The reconstruction of *spinal stability* is then a crucial step for the success of the operation. An *anterior fixation* (Fig. 12.5a, b) is mandatory to assure enough stability since when a second stage would be possible realizing 360 degrees stabilization. Meticulous attention is paid to detail, particularly during the mobilization of the posterior margins of the tumor which may be adherent to the dura. If the dura is torn, it should be immediately repaired.

12.1.5 Closure

A meticulous hemostasis must be performed with bipolar cautery, bone wax or other hemostatic

materials. It is so possible to close the posterior pharyngeal wall with interrupted 2-0 Vicryl sutures. A watertight closure must be secured to prevent leakage of saliva into the prevertebral space. Following closure of the pharyngeal wall, a nasogastric feeding tube can be introduced and the soft palate is approximated accurately in the midline in two layers with interrupted 3-0 Vicryl sutures. Our more recent experience has demonstrated the advantages of the percutaneous endoscopic gastrostomy (PEG) which is actually our preferred protocol to reduce local irritation and infection rate. The closure of the glossotomy is then accomplished in three layers. The deep layer of the intrinsic musculature is approximated from side-to-side to restore its anatomic continuity, while closure of the mucosa of the dorsum of the tongue is undertaken with interrupted 2-0 Vicryl sutures accurately aligning the two halves of the tongue, and particularly its tip. The closure continues on its ventral surface, on the anterior third and then the floor of the mouth up to the midline of the anterior gingiva. Accurate alignment of the two ends of the mandible at the osteotomy site must be secured in a stable way using two titanium miniplates. The skin incision of the lower lip and chin is closed in two

Fig. 12.5 a, b A direct visualization of the vertebral body associated with side to side control of the lesion and extended distally, facilitate spinal reconstruction with metal implants

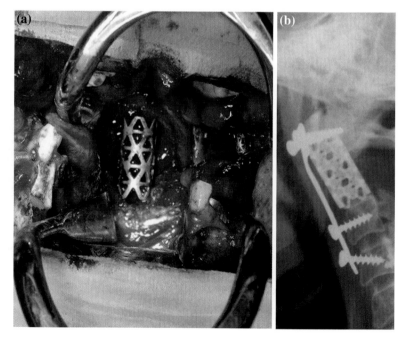

layers with 3-0 Vicryl in the deep one, and with 4-0 Nylon at the skin site, with accurate reapproximation of the vermilion border and the contour of the chin. Finally, a suction drain is brought out under the chin. Since the spinal stability was secured by means of an internal fixation, which can be extended down to the C4, in most of the cases, there is no need for an external brace. The transmandibular tongue-splitting approach allows for a clear visualization of the upper cervical spine and the clivus and offers an easy opportunity for a stable reconstruction.

Tumors are frequently located in the vertebral body and often near junctions. Therefore, it frequently is necessary to use a combined anteroposterior approach. Reconstructive surgery has a primary role in the treatment of spinal tumors. The instabilities at the craniocervical junction secondary to tumor resection represent a severe feature associated with life threatening risk. Residual instability requires a combined approach and internal fixation. Numerous internal fixation techniques exist for the craniovertebral junction, some of which involve screwplate fixation. Screw-plate fixation by Roy-Camille and developments of the Luque's

procedure (i.e., sublaminar wiring) led to the Hartshill technique and a modification, the Ransford loop and the posterior occipitocervical fusion (occiput-atlas-axis) using a "Y" plate as described by Grob. We designed a craniocervical fixation procedure using a cranial claw by hooks, which counteracts flexion/extension, lateral bending, axial rotation and shear forces. This metal construct is indicated in severe cases with significant bone destruction and high instability, such as tumoral osteolytic lesions [11]. The cranial claw with hooks is a stable anchor even in presence of osteopenic bone and can counteract the most severe stresses. It is of crucial importance the craniocervical angle of the fixation construct, and it is mandatory to avoid an anteversion of the occiput which can be responsible for severe complications.

12.2 Complications

These approaches are technically demanding and can be associated with cosmetic and functional complications. Crockard and Harms analyzed complication rates in a retrospective review of 97

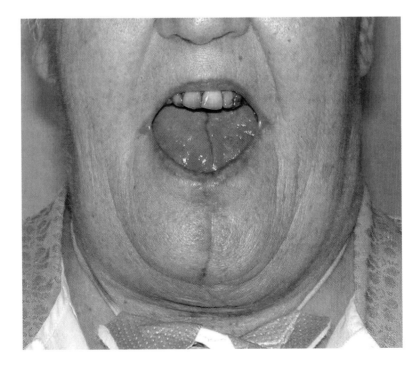

Fig. 12.6 Only minimal cosmetic impairment and functional disturbances experienced this female patient who survived 5 years pain free and without motor loss

patients treated with transoral, transfacial, transmandibular and anterior cervical approaches for resecting chordomas of the upper cervical spine and craniocervical junction. Dysphagia was more frequent with mandibulotomy and glossotomy, and this complication was not strictly associated with tracheostomy or occipitocervical fixation. In our series, we had a patient operated for primary tumor resection (chordoma), who died 16 days after the operation as a consequence of aortic dissection. Another patient was reoperated for a pressure sore of the posterior wall of the pharynx due to the nasogastric tube. All other patients underwent a PEG in the preoperative period. One patient experienced infection and was treated with antibiotics. One patient complained moderate transient dysphagia probably secondary to the glossotomy. The cosmetic impairment was minimized in males (Fig. 12.6) by coverage with a beard. Pull out of one anterior screw totally asymptomatic occurred in one case. Nerve palsy, intraoperative hemorrhage and cerebrospinal fluid leakage never occurred. The mandible osteotomy fixed with screw/plate fused in all cases.

12.3   Conclusion

The objectives of the surgical treatment of spinal non-traumatic lesions of the upper cervical spine are to palliate pain, restore or maintain neurological function and stabilize the spine. The improvement of diagnostic modalities, the development of new surgical approaches and more adequate fixation devices for anterior and posterior stabilization of the spine have led to treat the majority of the lesions. The transmandibular tongue-splitting approach is a useful procedure for treating primary and secondary lesions at the upper cervical spine with minor *cosmetic* and *functional impairment*. Combined internal fixation is often required. Stabilizing constructs must be resistant to relevant mechanical stresses and long lasting.

References

1. Fang HSY, Ong GB (1962) Direct anterior approach to the upper cervical spine. J Bone Joint Surg [AM] 44-A:1588–1604
2. Hodgson AR, Stock FE, Fang HS, Ong GB (1960) Anterior spinal fusion the operative approach and pathological findings in 412 patients with Pott's disease of the spine. Br J Surg 48:172–178
3. Logroscino CA (1989) Transoral surgery: a useful approach to the upper cervical spine. Springer, Berlin
4. Schmelzle R, Harms J (1984) Indication and limits of the transoral entry by treatment of fractures, luxation and tumors of the vertebral column. Presented at 7th congress of the European association for maxillo-facial surgery, Paris
5. Harms J, Schmelzle R, Stoltze D (1987) Osteosynthesen im occipito-cervicalen ubergang vom transoralen Zugang aus. In: 17th SICOT World Congress Abstracts Munich: Demeter Verlag
6. Schmelzle R, Harms J (1987) Craniocervical junction: diseases, diagnostic application of imaging procedures, surgical technics. Fortschr Kiefer Gesichtschir 32:206–208
7. Youssef AS, Guiot B, Black K, Sloan AE (2008) Modifications of the transoral approach to craniovertebral junction: anatomic study and clinical considerations. Neurosurgery 62(3 suppl 1): 145–155
8. James D, Crockard HA (1991) Surgical access to the base of the skull and upper cervical spine by extended maxillotomy. Neurosurgery 29:411–416
9. Hall JE, Denis F, Murray J (1977) Exposure of the upper cervical spine for spinal decompression by a mandible and tongue splitting approach. Case report. J Bone Joint Surg [Am] 55:121–123
10. Logroscino CA, Casula S, Rigante M, Almadori G (2004) Transmandible approach for the treatment of upper cervical spine metastatic tumors. Orthopedics 27(10):1100–1103
11. Logroscino CA, Diop A, Lavaste F (1996) Development of a new short metal construct for the treatment of severe craniovertebral instability: biomechanical evaluation. Spine State of the Art Reviews 10

Part IV

Infections

13

Stergios N. Lallos and Nikolaos E. Efstathopoulos

13.1 History: Epidemiology

Going back through the centuries, a skeleton from about 5000 BC was found to have spinal infection by tuberculosis [1]. Latter evidence of spinal infections was found in Egypt, in mummies from the Predynastic periods (3000 BC and earlier). In 1910, Ruffer reported the typical features of Pott's disease in an old Egyptian mummy Neshparenham, a priest of Amun (1000 BC, twenty-first Dynasty) [2]. Spinal deformities, very similar to those of Pott's disease were described by Hippocrates of Cos (460–375 BC) in his book entitled "On Articulations" [3] whereas bench stretching was suggested as treatment, a very popular intervention for a long time. Many centuries later, in 1896, the surgeon Jean-Francois Calot (1861–1944) described in a paper he read to the Academy of Medicine in Paris his technique entitled "redressment brusque" (or "redressment force") based on the Hippocratic procedure; the operation was named after him [4].

Despite the previous historical reports on the tuberculosis nature of spinal deformity by Hippocrates and Galen [5], it was Sir Percival Pott (1714–1788) in 1779, an English surgeon, who reported a systematic description of this spinal deformity (known as Pott's disease, there after), which became a historical paper for clinical practice [6]. Interestingly latter, there were cumulative reports on pyogenic infection of the spine [7] whereas at the end of the 19th century, the mortality rate of this condition in children and young adults was estimated as high as 70 % [8].

The incidence of vertebral osteomyelitis ranges from 0.5 to 2.2/100.000 inhabitants/year in two Scandinavian studies [9, 10]. Nonspecific vertebral osteomyelitis accounts for 3–4 % of all spinal infections whereas the cervical spine is affected in 3–10 % cases. The epidural abscess in this region is less common, estimated to occur in approximately 1/100.000 people [11]. Mortality caused by cervical spine osteomyelitis is considerable, and in case it is complicated by abscess, the morbidity and mortality remain higher [12, 13] with the latter to account for 15 % of all cases [14].

In vertebral osteomyelitis, there is high heterogeneity in the proportion of infection of the different parts of the spine, with the lumbar spine to be the predominant region that is affected. Regarding the cervical spine, isolated involvement of the atlantoaxial segment has rarely been documented in the English literature [15–28]. When the odontoid processes was affected by osteomyelitis, in some patients

S. N. Lallos (✉) · N. E. Efstathopoulos
Second Department of Orthopaedics, Athens
University Medical School Athens, Agias Olgas
Street 3-5, Nea Ionia, Attiki 14233, Greece
e-mail: st.lallos@gmail.com

N. E. Efstathopoulos
e-mail: nefstatho@med.uoa.gr

subsequent dislocation of the atlantoaxial joint [16, 25] or formation of epidural abscess with progressive neurological deficits was complicated [23, 26, 29]. Another rare clinical entity is infection of the occipitoatlantoaxial complex (septic arthritis of the facet joints) whereas Halla et al. [30] were the first who reported septic arthritis of the lateral facet joint combined with pseudo-Grisel's syndrome.

Osteomyelitis of the cervical spine, including the dens, in adults and particularly in the elderly may be hematogenous whereas in the majority it is attributed to direct extension from epidural, parapharyngeal or retropharyngeal abscess [22, 29, 31]. In children, there has been a paucity of reports of osteomyelitis of the atlas or axis. Today, spinal infections occur predominantly in the elderly; however, in young adults, it appears to have increased in recent decades because of immunodeficiency syndromes and intravenous drug abuse [32].

Regarding the epidemiology of the pathogenesis, it is well known that mycobacterium tuberculosis was the main reported pathogen in the first axis with destruction of the vertebra and formation of multiple prevertebral abscesses [33]. While in the developed world, spinal tuberculosis has become rare, the incidence seems to be increasing again because of immigrants, extensive tourism into developing countries and HIV infections [34–38]. In the past, tuberculosis has played an important role as a cause of spinal deformities and was one of the most common "orthopedic" diseases all over the world. Before antibiotics were available, 60 % of patients with neurological symptoms subsequent to tuberculous spondylitis died [39]. Nowadays, <5 % of similar affected patients die of the disease [40, 41], but spinal infection still can have devastating consequences. Despite the progress in the diagnosis and treatment of infectious disease that have improved the prognosis for patients with spinal infections, this medical condition remains a potentially life-threatening disease even in the industrialized world.

13.2 Clinical Presentation

13.2.1 Predisposing Factors

Hematogenous vertebral osteomyelitis may be caused by any condition that results in bacteremia. The infection spread through the bloodstream contaminating the venous plexus of the occipitocervical region and further the odontoid process. Infections of the urinary tract, soft tissue, or respiratory tract and intravenous drug abuse are all common causes. Poorly controlled diabetes mellitus, corticosteroids, aging, immunodeficiency, malnutrition, smoking, preoperative hospitalization, preexisting paraplegia, dental granulomas and previous septic conditions are all reported to predispose to spine osteomyelitis. In a large series of 854 patients with epidural spinal abscess, 377 had extra spinal focuses of infection [14] and 23 of these were diagnosed with urinary tract infections as the source of the abscess. Interestingly, patients with rheumatoid arthritis have high infection rate (5–18 %) [42–45], and the rate is even higher in Down syndrome population [46].

13.2.2 History of the Disease, Symptoms and Signs

The main problem in the management of patients with spinal infections is the delayed diagnosis. This is clearly presented in a literature review [47], in which only 20 % of patients had symptom duration of <3 weeks, 20 % had complaints for 3 weeks to 3 months and the remaining 50 % of individuals had symptoms for >3 months prior to diagnosis. In general, the history of patients with spinal infections is highly variable and non-specific unless neurological deficits are present. The clinical presentation is related to the virulence of the organism, immunocompetence of the host and duration of the infection and may be acute, subacute, or chronic. More than 90 % of patients, report a slowly progressive, continuous and localized neck pain, pain exacerbation at night and/or at rest and gibbus (in spinal tuberculosis). About 50 % of patients have fever which is more common in acute infections. When the infection is complicated by an epidural abscess, the patients occasionally complain of symptoms of radiculopathy and myelopathy. In about 15 % of cases, atypical symptoms such as meningeal irritation, headache, chest pain or respiratory problems may occur. Neurological deficits occur in a rate of 17 % of all patients with vertebral osteomyelitis. The rate is higher in cervical lesions. Stone et al. [48] showed that more than half their patient with cervical infection had neurological deficits. Less common findings may be muscle spasm, tenderness, weight loss, "feeling sick," pain exacerbation with movement and weight bearing and limited motion.

Focusing on infection of cervical spine, Zigler et al. [28] described the difficulties a clinician is faced for the diagnosis of this disease due to the atypical clinical presentation. For early diagnosis of the disease, a rarely presented triad of elevated temperature, neck pain and progressive neurological deficit may be helpful [49]. Other early signs and symptoms as cervical spine lymphadenopathy, spasm of neck musculature and progressive torticollis followed by subfebrility have been described for upper cervical spine infections [16]. In a case study of Busche et al. [16], the authors described a young man with diabetes mellitus and some of the later mentioned symptoms in the upper cervical spine of 6-month duration before a sudden change for the worse. In line was the case of an elderly patient described by Noguchi et al. [23] who complained of neck pain and stiffness for 7 days and had symptoms of meningeal irritation. CT and MRI scans revealed odontoid osteomyelitis and abscess formation.

In the same context, osteomyelitis of the odontoid process is a rare disease that is often difficult to diagnose. The initial presenting symptoms can be non-specific, and definitive neurological signs develop relatively late in the disease. An afebrile, non-toxic-appearing pediatric patient with persistent neck stiffness or torticollis may have acute osteomyelitis of the odontoid process. In a case report, an 18-month-old boy who had been treated for a cutaneous abscess presented to the emergency room for neck stiffness, malaise and anorexia. The boy was afebrile with a normal peripheral blood cell count but an elevated erythrocyte sedimentation rate. However, a non-contrast CT scan showed destructive changes throughout the odontoid process, and the body of C2 and a magnetic resonance image confirmed abnormal enhancement of the odontoid process and thickening of the prevertebral soft tissues [50]. The diagnosis might be more obscure given the uncommon location of the infection; a case of isolated tuberculous involvement of the spinous process of the axis, presenting as a posterior cervical lump in the absence of disease process in any other part of the body [51].

Therefore, as already mentioned, osteomyelitis of the spine requires a high index of suspicion for the diagnosis. In addition to that, several factors contribute to the difficulty in diagnosing infection of some spinal regions such the atlantoaxial [52]. The anatomy of the atlantoaxial articulation is different from other segments of the spinal column. The atlantoaxial joint consists primarily of synovial joints with no disks between the two adjacent vertebrae. The infection often starts as septic arthritis. The narrowing disk space, usually evident in early osteomyelitis of the spine, is not seen, and radiographic changes are frequently not evident until late in the disease process. In addition, widening of the retropharyngeal soft tissue is easily missed, especially by inexperienced practitioners. Given these additional reasons, clinicians should be very careful and highly suspicious. Delay in diagnosis can be catastrophic with development of an epidural abscess and consequent death or major neurological disability.

13.3 Diagnostic Workout

The key to diagnosis is the clinical suspicion of spinal infection. Neither blood test is specific for the diagnosis; however, CRP and ESR are almost always elevated while the white blood cell count can remain normal especially in chronic infections. ESR is increased in >90 % of patients; however, because of its low specificity, it is usually used to check treatment response. CRP has advantages over the ESR in the evaluation and follow-up of patients with spinal infection because the level increases more rapidly and has a much shorter half-life.

13.4 Imaging

In spinal osteomyelitis, radiographic changes cannot usually be identified until there is advanced osseous destruction; therefore, the introduction and development of CT and MRI have simplified the diagnostic procedure in the recent decades [30]. The major drawback of standard radiography is the delay of radiological signs up to 2–4 weeks after the onset of the disease. The main findings are blurred endplates, disk space collapse, development of osteolysis and a paravertebral shadow, and late changes such as reactive bone formation, fracture and kyphotic deformity (Fig. 13.1). Progressively, infection may extend to adjacent levels. Lateral films are useful to visualize the prevertebral soft tissue swelling that is characteristic of cervical osteomyelitis and one of the earliest signs seen in addition to periosteal thickening or elevation and focal osteopenia. Prevertebral soft tissue swelling is usually due to edema caused by a near-by infection of the cervical spine or retropharyngeal abscess. Given the low cost and the wide availability of the plain films of the cervical spine, they should be performed initially. However, the early signs can be obscure and easily missed by an inexperienced radiologist, so other imaging modalities are obtained to aid in the early diagnosis of odontoid osteomyelitis.

Use of CT scan may be helpful to distinguish infection from malignancy and clearly demonstrate the extent of bony destruction and the formation of soft tissue abscesses. CT of the cervical spine allows for cross-sectional imaging of the atlantoaxial joint and surrounding tissues with reformatted coronal and sagittal views. CT is particularly useful to locate areas of periosteal reaction, cortical bone destruction and sequestrum or involucrum formation. CT is also reported to be more sensitive for the localization of bone sequestration than MRI [53]. Contrast

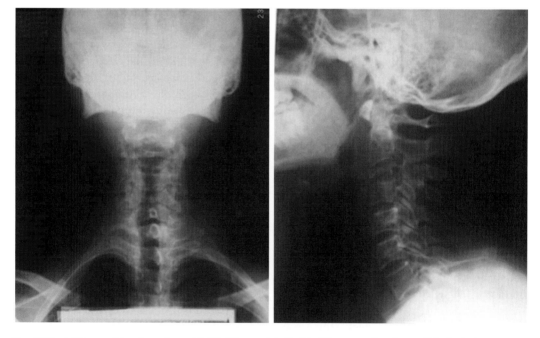

Fig. 13.1 A 33-year-old male patient with C2–C3 spondylodiscitis (Courtesy of professor G.S. Sapkas)

images obtained with soft tissue window settings can detect associated prevertebral soft tissue swelling and delineation of rim-enhancing abscesses [54]. It is possible for adjacent soft tissue swelling to be apparent on CT before it is seen on plain films, as noted in the case by Limbird et al. [22] in which erosion of the odontoid process with adjacent soft tissue swelling was seen despite normal cervical plain films.

MRI is the imaging method of choice; it allows early diagnosis of infection and recognition of abscess formation (Fig. 13.2). It provides much more anatomic information than radionuclide studies, and results become positive at about the same time as a Gallium bone scan. MRI has 96 % sensitivity, 93 % specificity and 94 % accuracy in detecting vertebral osteomyelitis. Characteristic

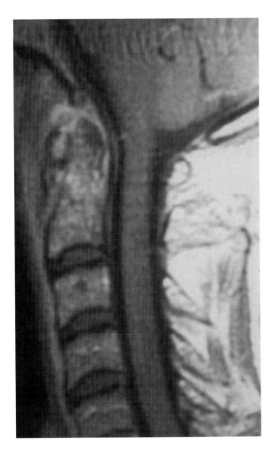

Fig. 13.2 MRI shows involvement of the axis and the prevertebral abscess due to Staphylococcus infection (Courtesy of professor G.S. Sapkas)

findings include decreased vertebral endplate signal intensity on T1-weighted images, loss of endplate definition, increased signal intensity on T2-weighted images and contrast enhancement of the disk and vertebral endplates. The enhanced images may distinguish active infections from those responding to treatment. In almost all cases, MRI distinguishes tumor from infection. MRI was the ideal method for providing quantitative view of the extent of neural compression, thereby allowing for an adequate determination of therapeutic options [52]. MRI is the method of choice for the early diagnosis of odontoid osteomyelitis [23, 31, 51]. Early in the course of odontoid osteomyelitis, changes consistent with uncomplicated osteomyelitis are visible on T1- and T2-weighted MR images; however, it is difficult to delineate between normal and abnormal bone marrow [55]. Short tau inversion recovery (STIR) and chemical fat-saturated post-contrast sequences readily reveal intraosseous abnormal signal or enhancement and should be used in MRI protocols to rule out marrow involvement and/or an epidural abscess early in the course of the disease [53, 55].

Radionuclide studies allow detection of spinal infections earlier than plain radiographs. Technetium-99-m-labeled methylene-diphosphonate (Tc-99 m MDP) bone scintigraphy is currently infrequently used for the diagnosis of spinal infections (Fig. 13.3). However, an indication for a bone scan is still the search for a focus lesion, for example, dental granuloma and osteomyelitis. Gallium scan shows evidence of infection earlier in the course of the disease than 99 m-Tc scans, appears normal during resolution of the infection and had slightly higher specificity than Tc scans.

Confusion may arise in differentiating spinal infection from disk degeneration. Positron from infection emission tomography (PET) with fluorine-18 fluorodeoxyglucose (FDG) has been shown to be helpful. [18F]-FDG PET appears to be especially helpful in those cases in which MRI cannot be performed or is non-diagnostic and as an adjunct in patients in whom the diagnosis is inconclusive [56]. Prompt diagnosis is facilitated by early and appropriate imaging techniques. However, despite the accuracy of

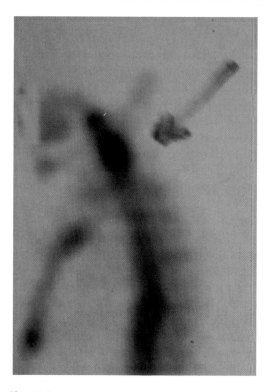

Fig. 13.3 99 m-Tc bone scan shows increased radio-isotope uptake at the upper cervical spine (Courtesy of professor G.S. Sapkas)

Proteus) which are common causes of urinary tract infections, Pseudomonas aeruginosa (in 65 % of drug abusers), *Streptococcus viridians* and *Propionibacterium acnes*. Anaerobic infections are uncommon and generally are associated with open fractures, infected wounds, human bites, foreign bodies or diabetes mellitus. Salmonella species osteomyelitis is encountered rarely and has a tendency to infect sites of pre-existing disease. Reports for coagulase-negative Staphylococcus are very rare causative pathogens of spinal infection. Hadjipavlou et al. [62] reviewed 34 patients with spinal infection treated with surgical percutaneous transpedicular drainage, and found positive cultures in 73.5 % out of which 16 % cases of coagulase-negative Staphylococcus. A meta-analysis of 915 patients with spinal epidural abscesses [14] confirmed the pathogen in 753 cases, and only in 35, the etiological factor was coagulase-negative Staphylococcus species. A case of polymicrobial osteomyelitis of the odontoid process with epidural abscess, caused by a synergistic infection with Staphylococcus aureus and Proteus mirabilis, was also reported [31].

MRI, an absolute diagnosis must be based on bacteriologic or histologic examination of the pathologic tissue [57, 58].

13.5 Biopsy

The isolation of the causative organism is very important and must be attempted in every case. Biopsy under CT guidance is preferable because of the accurate spatial resolution, which is important to document that the biopsy was actually taken from within the lesion. This is particularly precious in areas that are difficult to access, such as the upper cervical region [59]. Percutaneous needle biopsy provides a definitive diagnosis ranging from 57 to 92 % [59–61] depending on previous administration of antibiotics (Fig. 13.4).

The most frequently found microorganism is Staphylococcus aureus (30–35 %), gram-negative pathogens (*E. coli*, Enterococcus and

13.6 Treatment

The goals of treatment are to establish the diagnosis, prevent or reverse neurological deficits, establish spinal stability, eradicate the infection, relieve pain and prevent any possible relapse. The optimal antibiotic therapy plays the key role in the treatment of spinal infections. Regarding the cervical spine infections, there have a higher risk of complication and surgical treatment is often required as adjunct to antibiotics.

13.6.1 Conservative Treatment

The majority of patients can be successfully treated non-operatively. The main indications for non-operative treatment are known causative microorganism, absence of gross bony destruction and instability, absence of relevant

Fig. 13.4 CT-guided biopsy (Courtesy of professor G.S. Sapkas)

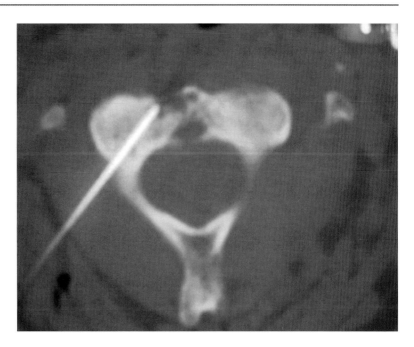

neurological deficit, rapid normalization of inflammation parameters and mobile patients with only moderate pain. Intravenous antibiotics for a minimum of 4–6 weeks, depending on the extent of the infection and the species of the organisms, are recommended as the gold standard for the treatment of bacterial and parasitic infections. The treatment success should be monitored by regular determination of the inflammation indices (white blood cell count, ESR and CRP). Antibiotic treatment should only be stopped after normalization of the CRP. In the case of persistent symptoms and non-decreasing inflammation parameters, imaging studies should be done.

The optimal antibiotic therapy should be guided by the biopsy result, the resistance of the organism and the bone penetration of the antibiotic. Antibiotics combined with occipitocervical immobilization have been reported to provide satisfactory outcome without recourse to surgical decompression and fixation [23, 63]. There is still debate on the optimal duration of the antituberculous chemotherapy required for complete recovery. A minimum of 12 months is favored by the majority of experts depending on the resistance and side effects [37]. Additionally,

upper cervical infections such as infections of the axis require a halo vest to control pain and to prevent deformity or neurological deterioration. When there is no evidence for instability, it was reported that early conservative treatment of atlantoaxial infection with antibiotics, immobilization and drainage of pus correlated with good outcomes [19, 21, 23, 29].

It is a matter of debate the treatment of complicated odontoid osteomyelitis with abscess formation. Successful clinical outcomes were reported in patients with vertebral osteomyelitis treated without surgery, especially in its early phase, when the segment is still stable [64]. However, successful outcomes were also reported in numerous recent studies by using operative treatment [28]. The presence of neurological findings indicates progressive cervical spine myelopathy and urgent surgical decompression is required. Thus, the success of treatment of infectious lesions in the upper cervical spine region is greatly dependent on the early diagnosis and initiation of therapy. However, once progressive paralysis occurs, operative decompression should be performed, and if significant instability remains, surgical stabilization should be considered [16, 22, 25–28]. Further indication for a change from non-operative to operative treatment is the persistence of the infection despite adequate antibiotic treatment or in the presence of drug side effects limiting the further use of specific antibiotics in adequate dosage.

13.7 Operative Treatment

About one-third of patients with spinal infections need operative treatment. The major indications for operative treatment are disease progression despite adequate antibiotic treatment, neurological compromise, progressive spinal deformity, instability and incapacitating pain and severe abscess. The surgical approach depends on the extent and location of the infection, spinal destruction, neurological deficits, health status and comorbidity of the patient. A single-stage anterior approach is best suited for cases in the absence of gross deformity or instability, predominant anterior column involvement and effective radical debridement. Transoral decompressive surgery is well described for the treatment of the odontoid osteomyelitis and is both safe and effective [18, 65]. However, it does require particular surgical and anesthetic expertise as well as specialized instrumentation [66, 67]. The posterior approach is a safe alternative in an emergency for surgeons less familiar with the transoral approach.

The surgical options are radical debridement; radical debridement and bone grafting; and radical debridement, bone grafting and instrumentation. Radical debridement and bone grafting are indicated in patients with intravertebral abscess and without gross bony destruction, deformity and instability. In many cases, additional spinal stabilization is required. Instrumentation is still controversial, but growing evidence has shown that implants can be used without side effects [68]. Spinal instrumentation promotes rather than prevents resolution of the infection because of the added stability. Implants can be used at the site of infection in the cervical spine with the prerequisite that radical debridement is thoroughly achieved.

Osteomyelitis of the axis is rare and often difficult to diagnose. In the presence of the triad of neck pain, and fever with or without neurological symptoms and signs, the possibility of osteomyelitis should be considered, particularly in immunocompromised patients. MRI provides for early diagnosis of a potentially life-threatening condition [23, 26, 69]. High-dose, broad-spectrum, empirical antibiotic therapy should be administered, pending the results of the culture and the bacteriological sensitivities. In adjunct, rigid occipitocervical immobilization or surgical stabilization may be needed. In selected patients, surgical decompression of the cervico-medullary junction is necessary, safe and effective. Early and optimal treatment is the mainstay of management and is associated with a favorable prognosis [18, 26, 29, 69].

References

1. Tate J (1966) Sjukdomarnas historia ochgeografi, Stockholm, Albers BonniersForläg. Longmanns Green, London (English trans.)
2. Ruffer MA (1918) Arthritis deformans and spondylitis in ancient Egypt. J Pathol Bacteriol 22: 212–226
3. Capps E, Page TE, Rouse WHD (1927) Hippocrates: on joints. In: Withington ET (ed) Hippocrates: the loeb classical library, vol 3. W. Heinemann, London, pp 200–397
4. Mounier-Kuhn A, Sutter B (2005) François Calot's concepts about the treatment of osteoarticular tuberculosis (in French). Hist Sci Med 39(3):303–314
5. Kuhn CG (1964) Galen: De usupartium-corporishumani. In: ClaudiiGaleni Opera Omnia, vol 4, Georg Olms, Hildesheim, pp 42–119
6. Pott P (1779) Remarks on that kind of palsy of the lower limbs which is frequently found to accompany a curvature of the spine. Johnson, London
7. Lannelongue OM (1897) On acute osteomyelitis. Miscellaneous, Pathological and Practical Medicine Tracts, Paris
8. Makins GH, Abbott FC (1896) On acute primary osteomyelitis of the vertebrae. Ann Sur 23(5): 510–539
9. Beronius M, Bergman B, Anderson R (2001) Vertebral osteomyelitis in Goteborg, Sweden: a retrospective study of patients during 1990–1995. Scand J Infect Dis 33:527–532
10. Krogsgaard MR, Wagn P, Bengtsson J (1998) Epidemiology of acute vertebral osteomyelitis in Denmark: 137 cases in Denmark 1978–1982,

compared to cases reported to the National Patient Register 1991–1993. Acta Orthop Scand 69(5): 513–517

11. Acosta FL, Chin CT, Quinones-Hinojosa A, Ames C, Weinstein PR, Chou D (2004) Diagnosis and management of adult pyogenic osteomyelitis of the cervical spine. Neurosurg Focus 17:1–9

12. Hlavin ML, Kaminski HJ, Ross JS, Ganz E (1990) Spinal epidural abscess: a ten-year perspective. Neurosurgery 27(2):177–184

13. Lu CH, Chang WN, Lui CC, Lee PY, Chang HW (2002) Adult spinal epidural abscess: clinical features and prognostic factors. Clin Neurol Neurosurg 104(4):306–310

14. Reihsaus E, Waldbaur H, Seeling W (2000) Spinal epidural abscess: a meta-analysis of 915 patients. Neurosurg Rev 232:175–204

15. Anton K, Christoph R, Cornelius FM (1999) Osteomyelitis and pathological fracture of the axis. Case illustration. J Neurosurg 90:162

16. Busche M, Bastian L, Riedemann NC et al (2005) Complete osteolysis of the dens with atlantoaxial luxation caused by infection with Staphylococcus aureus. Spine 30:369–374

17. Fukutake T, Kitazaki H, Hattori T (1998) Odontoid osteomyelitis complicating pneumococcal pneumonia. EurNeurol 39:126–127

18. Keogh S, Crockard A (1992) Staphylococcal infection of the odontoid peg. Postgrad Med J 68: 51–54

19. Kubo S, Takimoto H, Hosoi K et al (2002) Osteomyelitis of the odontoid process associated with meningitis and retropharyngeal abscess-case report. Neurol Med Chir 42:447–451

20. Kurimoto M, Endo S, Ohi M et al (1998) Pyogenic osteomyelitis of an invaginated odontoid process with rapid deterioration of high cervical myelopathy: a case report. Acta Neurochir 140:1093–1094

21. Leach RE, Goldstein HH, Younger D (1967) Osteomyelitis of the odontoid process. A case report. J Bone Joint Surg Am 49:369–371

22. Limbird TJ, Brick GW, Boulas HJ et al (1988) Osteomyelitis of the odontoid process. J Spinal Disord 1:66–74

23. Noguchi S, Yanaka K, Yamada Y et al (2000) Diagnostic pitfalls in osteomyelitis of the odontoid process: case report. Surg Neurol 53:573–578

24. Ruskin J, Shapiro S, McCombs M et al (1992) Odontoid osteomyelitis. An unusual presentation of an uncommon disease. West J Med 156:306–308

25. Suchomel P, Buchvald P, Barsa P et al (2003) Pyogenic osteomyelitis of the odontoid process: single stage decompression and fusion. Spine 28: 239–244

26. Wiedau-Pazos M, Curio G, Grusser C (1999) Epidural abscess of the cervical spine with osteomyelitis of the odontoid process. Spine 24: 133–136

27. Venger BH, Musher DM, Brown EW et al (1986) Isolated C-2 osteomyelitis of hematogenous origin: case report and literature review. Neurosurgery 18: 461–464

28. Zigler JE, Bohlman HH, Robinson RA et al (1987) Pyogenic osteomyelitis of the occiput, the atlas, and the axis. A report of five cases. J Bone Joint Surg Am 69:1069–1073

29. Young WF, Weaver M (1999) Isolated pyogenic osteomyelitis of the odontoid process. Scand J Infect Dis 31:512–515

30. Halla JT, Bliznak JG, Finn S (1991) Septic arthritis of the C1–C2 lateral facet joint and torticollis: pseudo-Grisel's syndrome. Arthritis Rheum 34:84–88

31. Haridas A, Walsh DC, Mowle DH (2003) Polymicrobial osteomyelitis of the odontoid process with epidural abscess: case report and review of literature. Skull Base 13:107–111

32. Jellis JE (1995) Bacterial infections: bone and joint tuberculosis. Baillieres Clin Rheumatol 9:151–159

33. Lindquist SW, Steinmetz BA, Starke JR (1997) Multidrug-resistant tuberculosis of the first cervical vertebra in an immunocompetent adolescent. Pediatr Infect Dis J 16:333–336

34. Barnes PF, Bloch AB, Davidson PT, Snider DE Jr (1991) Tuberculosis in patients with human immunodeficiency virus infection. N Engl J Med 324(23):1644–1650

35. Brancker A (1991) Tuberculosis in Canada, 1989. Health Rep 3(1):92–96

36. Halsey JP, Reeback JS, Barnes CG (1982) A decade of skeletal tuberculosis. Ann Rheum Dis 41(1):7–10

37. Pertuiset E, Beaudreuil J, Lioté F et al (1999) Spinal tuberculosis in adults. A study of 103 cases in a developed country, 1980–1994. Medicine 78(5): 309–320

38. Rieder HL, Cauthen GM, Kelly GD et al (1989) Tuberculosis in the United States. JAMA 262(3): 385–389

39. Bosworth DM, Della Pietra A, Rahilly G (1953) Paraplegia resulting from tuberculosis of the spine. J Bone Joint Surg Am 35(3):735–740

40. Adendorff JJ, Boeke EJ, Lazarus C (1987) Tuberculosis of the spine: results of management of 300 patients. J R Coll Surg Edinb 32(3):152–155

41. Lifeso RM, Weaver P, Harder EH (1985) Tuberculous spondylitis in adults. J Bone Joint Surg Am 67(9):1405–1413

42. Santavirta S, Slatis P, Kankaapaa U et al (1988) Treatment of the cervical spine in rheumatoid arthritis. J Bone Joint Surg Am 70:658–667

43. Wertheim SB, Bohlmann HH (1987) Occipitocervical fusion: indications, technique, and long-term results in thirteen patients. J Bone Joint Surg Am 69:833–836

44. Clark CR, Goetz DD, Menezes AH (1989) Arthrodesis of the cervical spine in rheumatoid arthritis. J Bone Joint Surg Am 71:381–392

45. Bryan WJ, Inglis AE, Sculco TP et al (1982) Methylmethacrylate stabilization for enhancement of posterior cervical arthrodesis in rheumatoid arthritis. J Bone Joint Surg 64:1045–1050

46. Segal LS, Drummond DS, Zanotti RM et al (1991) Complications of posterior arthrodesis of the cervical spine in patients who have Down syndrome. J Bone Joint Surg Am 73:1547–1554

47. Sapico FL, Montgomerie JZ (1990) Vertebral osteomyelitis. Infect Dis Clin North Am 4(3): 539–550

48. Stone JL, Cybulski GR, Rodriguez J, Gryfinski ME, Kant R (1989) Anterior cervical debridement and strut-grafting for osteomyelitis of the cervical spine. J Neurosurg 70(6):879–883

49. Ross J, Brant-Zawadzki M, Chen M, Moore K, Salzman K (2004) Diagnostic imaging: spine, 1st edn. Amirsys, Altona, pp 1–14

50. Nolting L, Singer J, Hackett R, Kleiner L (2010) Acute hematogenous osteomyelitis of the odontoid process in a child with torticollis. PediatrEmer Care 26:669–671

51. Shamim MS et al (2009) Isolated tuberculosis of C2 spinous process. Spine 9:30–32

52. Gormley W, Rock J (1994) Spontaneous atlantoaxial osteomyelitis: no longer a rare case? Case report. Neurosurgery 35:133–136

53. Marin C, Sanchez-Alegre M et al (2004) Magnetic resonance imaging of osteoarticular infections in children. Curr Probl Radiol 33:43–59

54. Oudjhane K, Azouz E (2001) Imaging of osteomyelitis in children. Radiol Clin North Am 39:251–266

55. Schmit P, Glorion C (2004) Osteomyelitis in infants and children. Eur Radiol 14:L44–L54

56. Gemmel F, Rijk PC, Collins JM, Parlevliet T, Stumpe KD, Palestro CJ (2010) Expanding role of 18F-fluoro-D-deoxyglucose PET and PET/CT in spinal infections. Eur Spine J 19(4):540–551

57. An HS, Seldomridge JA (2006) Spinal infections: diagnostic tests and imaging studies. Clin Orthop Relat Res 444:27–33

58. Tyrrell PN, Cassar-Pullicino VN, McCall IW (1999) Spinal infection. Eur Radiol 9:1066–1077

59. Omarini LP, Garcia J (1993) CT-guided percutaneous puncture-biopsy of the spine. Review of 104 cases. Schweiz Med Wochenschr 123(46):2191–2197

60. Brugières P, Gaston A, Voisin MC, Ricolfi F, Chakir N (1992) CT-guided percutaneous biopsy of the cervical spine: a series of 12 cases. Neuroradiology 34(4):358–360

61. Rieneck K, Hansen SE, Karle A, Gutschik E (1996) Microbiologically verified diagnosis of infectious spondylitis using CT-guided fine needle biopsy. APMIS 104:755–762

62. Hadjipavlou AG, Katonis PK, Gaitanis IN, Muffoletto AJ, Tzermiadianos MN, Crow W (2004) Percutaneous transpedicular discectomy and drainage in pyogenic spondylodiscitis. Eur Spine J 13: 707–713

63. Azizi SA, Fayad PB, Fulbright R, Giroux ML, Waxman SG (1995) Clivus and cervical spinal osteomyelitis with epidural abscess presenting with multiple cranial neuropathies. Clin Neurol Neurosurg 97:239–244

64. SaSaki K, Nabeshima Y, Ozaki A, Mori H, Fuji H, Sumi M et al (2006) Septic arthritis of the atlantoaxial joint. Case report. J Spinal Disord Tech 19:612–615

65. Kanaan IU, Ellis M, Safi T, Al Kawi MZ, Coates R (1999) Craniocervical junction tuberculosis: a rare but dangerous disease. Surg Neurol 51:21–25

66. Jain VK, Behari S, Banerji D, Bhargava V, Chhabra DK (1999) Transoral decompression for craniovertebral osseous anomalies: perioperative management dilemmas. Neurol India 47:188–195

67. Knutti O, Kaech DL (1997) Postoperative high cervical quadriplegia after transoral biopsy of a paravertebral tuberculous abscess with epidural extension: complete resolution after decompressive laminectomy and high-dose methylprednisolone. Acta Neurochir 139:158–159

68. Faraj AA, Webb JK (2000) Spinal instrumentation for primary pyogenic infection report of 31 patients. Acta Orthop Belg 66(3):242–247

69. Fischer U, Vosshenrich R (1990) Osteomyelitis (spinal infection, spondylitis, spondylodiscitis) of the dens axis. Rontgenblatter 43:54–57

Congenital Malformations

14

Carlos Villas

14.1 Knowledge on the Malformations of the Axis. Why May be Interesting?

Congenital malformations of the occipitocervical junctional region are very rare in daily practice. Nevertheless, despite they are seldom and briefly reported in specialized books [1–6] (a single page in the super-specialized one by Mallet et Lechevalier) [6, 7] or papers (most of times on a case), its knowledge is not anecdotic and it is obliged for doctors devoted to cervical spine conditions. Frequently, differential diagnosis may be difficult in case of trauma. As referred to by Shapiro et al. [8], "Nothing is more confusing (either to the resident in the emergency room at 3:00 A.M., or to the attending radiologist later in the day) than a myriad of poorly exposed, poorly positioned views of the atlanto-axial joints. Fracture or no fracture? Subluxation or no subluxation? Normal or abnormal?" Remnant normal non-ossified synchondroses or aberrant ossification centers must be differentiated from *fracture* lines or traumatic fragmentation [8].

The natural history of some congenital malformations of the axis is uncertain, unpredictable, and often leads to lifetime wearing a brace for the fear of trauma, or a stabilizing operation by atlantoaxial fusion. Indeterminacy on the possibly devastating effect on normal life activities or after a trauma leads normally to take decisions looking for a definitive solution [9, 10].

14.1.1 Signs and Symptoms

Local stiffness or instability are the usual complaints, as in other disorders of the upper cervical spine [3]. When limited to one or two mobile segments, stiffness may be long time asymptomatic because of compensation by the adjacent segments but it may determine (normally at long term) degeneration of the compensating mobile segments; this degeneration may also cause pain/spasm and—associated to a narrow canal—may lead to cord compression resulting in progressive spondylotic myelopathy or acute cord damage. Instability may also cause pain/spasm and myelopathy due to repeated micro-trauma and direct compression in case of resulting subluxation or dislocation.

Painful complaints are normally referred to the occiput or the occipitocervical junction and they may appear spontaneously or after a trauma. Cord compression symptoms are normally related to the severity of the anomaly and the resulting instability. Neurological symptoms may be observed in children or adults, spontaneously or after a trauma—even minor—and range from

C. Villas (✉)
Orthopaedic Surgery and Traumatology, University of Navarre Clinic, Avda Pío XII 36, 31008, Pamplona, Spain
e-mail: cvillas@unav.es

D. S. Korres (ed.), *The Axis Vertebra*,
DOI: 10.1007/978-88-470-5232-1_14, © Springer-Verlag Italia 2013

slight sensory alterations or easy fatigability to quadriparesis, with a wide variety of clinical pictures.

14.1.2 Diagnosis

Present options given by image studies make diagnosis and definition of the congenital abnormalities easy today. Nevertheless, most of times we notice their existence with radiographs, CT scans or MRI in studies performed fortuitously—at random—or, more frequently, when studying patients who consult because of neck deformity (short neck, torticollis or facial deformity), cervical pain or/and neurological symptoms due to malalignment or instability. Although standard studies are diagnostic in many cases [8, 11], three-dimensional and multiplanar reformatted computed tomography have proved to be highly efficient by allowing a better definition of congenital anomalies of the upper cervical spine [12] (Fig. 14.1). For patients having contra-indication or obstacles to undergo a CT scan or MRI study, laminagrams

taken by lineal tomography are still a useful tool to bring a correct diagnosis (Fig. 14.2).

Congenital abnormalities are also frequently found in asymptomatic people when making general radiological screening studies which may be indicated in children with bone dysplasias (Morquio's syndrome or spondyloepiphyseal dysplasia, for example) polimalformative syndromes or Down's syndrome, cases in which congenital malformations of the upper cervical spine are likely to exist [13, 14].

14.1.3 Treatment

Therapeutic indication for atlantoaxial instability use to be a C1−C2 fusion, which may be extended cephalad to the occiput or more caudally depending on the specific anomaly and the exact localization of the instability. Cord compression at C1−C2 level may be treated by re-alignment of C1 on C2 in case of mobile subluxation or dislocation and by resection of the posterior arch of the atlas in the case of a rigid subluxation or dislocation. Pre-operative

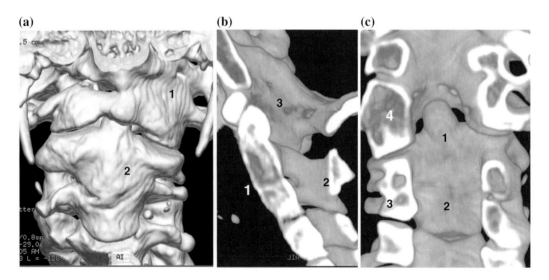

(a)   **(b)**   **(c)**

Fig. 14.1 a Frontal view of a 3D CT scan of the cervical spine with assimilation of the atlas. There is a visible OC1 synostosis on its *left side* (*1*) and a C2−C3 fusion, more evident at the *left side* of the vertebral body (*2*), **b** Lateral view showing fusion of the body (*1*) and the articular processes (*2*), the atlanto-occipital fusion being evident (*3*), **c** Hypoplasia of the odontoid process (*1*) and fusion od the body (*2*) and pedicles (*3*) in a posterior view, the atlanto-occipital fusion being also evident (*4*)

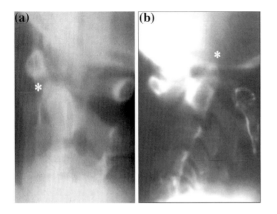

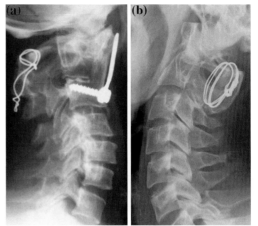

Fig. 14.2 a Lineal tomogram shows a small promontory at the base of an absent odontoid process (*star*) but also a small thinny-corticated os odontoideum, **b** Lineal tomogram shows a total C1−C2 dislocation and tetraparesis in a patient with Down's syndrome. The odontoid process appears in the *middle* of the foramen magnum (*star*)

Fig. 14.3 Lateral view of two patients who had C1−C3 and C1−C2 fusion 23 and 21 years before. **a** Patient affected of Down's syndrome. Operated twice at the age of 10 and 11 by posterior approach. Re-operated at the age of 12 with a C1−C3 fusion by anterior approach, the patient showed degenerative changes at different levels below the fusion at the age of 35. The fact that aging is usually precocious in people with Down's syndrome has to be considered. **b** Patient affected of os odontoideum with instability operated on at the age of 13. No degenerative changes are observed at the age of 33

reduction may be attempted by halo-traction or a similar procedure. Specially in children, surgery of the upper cervical spine is not free of obstacles, hazards and complications, the incidence of pseudarthrosis being non negligible.

Among the different options for O−C2 or C1−C2 stabilization (wires or rods connected to hooks or screws [9, 13, 15–17]) C1−C2 transarticular screws or constructs using rods connected to screws seem to provide the more efficient stabilization. Screws may be placed through the articular process of C1 and trough the pedicle, the laminae or the articular processes of C2. As an alternative, hooks may also serve to connect the rods., Nevertheless, we have to take into account that sometimes the pedicle of C2 is narrow and may not admit a screw in children or adults, specially when there exist dysplastic or elongated pedicles, C1−C2 subluxation or dislocation, or the anatomy is severely altered in some cases of polimaformative syndromes or generalized disorders of the skeleton. Furthermore, immature spines with poor development due to age or malformation of the posterior arch of the atlas [18, 19] may rend impossible the use of wires or hooks and sometimes may oblige to extend the fusion to the occiput. In case of surgery for fusion, absence of the posterior arch of the atlas may also rend more risky the posterior approach because of the possibility of entering the canal with instruments as Cobb elevators, for example.

Although adjacent problems would be reasonably expected after a C1−C2 fusion, specially in children, long-term outcome of patients having a C1−C2 arthrodesis is very good. There is a real paucity of reports of single cases or series with long follow-up and a negative outcome and we have good experience in children operated under the age of 14 and having 20 years of follow-up [20]. Only one patient with Down' syndrome and a C1−C3 fusion shoved signs of cervical spine degeneration from C3 to C7, but we have to consider that aging may be very precocious in this kind of patients [21] (Fig. 14.3). The possibility of obtaining a non-desired "hyper-arthrodesis", even with a careful approach has to be taken into account in young patients (Fig. 14.4). Even in these cases, the long term outcome is usually good, free of symptoms or complications.

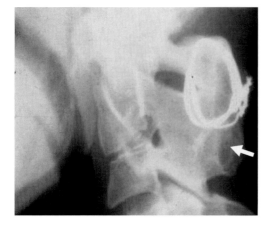

Fig. 14.4 Spontaneous—non desired—C2–C3 posterior fusion (*arrow*) in a case of C1–C2 arthrodesis as treatment of a C1–C2 instability due to os odontoideum

Degeneration adjacent to C2–C3 congenital fusion (at C3–C4 level) is not so frequent but—being symptomatic—may be treated by C3–C4 fusion or, depending on the degree of degeneration, by means of an arthroplasty with total disc prosthesis [17].

14.2 Embryology of the Axis Focused on Congenital Malformations

The time to start developing defects of segmentation—individualization among the adjacent vertebrae—or anomalous formation or fusion of the different parts or nuclei of a particular vertebra are between the fourth and the eighth weeks of foetal life. In this period, the membranous vertebral column is substituted by a cartilaginous one at and the vertebral arches start to ossify [4, 22–26].

Defects of segmentation-individualization will affect the relationship of the axis with the basal lamina (tip of the odontoid process), the atlas and the third cervical vertebra.

Failure of formation of the secondary nuclei may collaborate in the development of anomalies at the transverse processes and the tip of the odontoid, which sometimes develops independently as a small accessory bone separated from

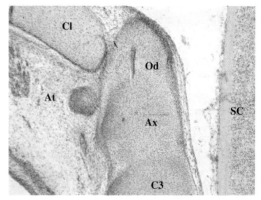

Fig. 14.5 Sagittal section of a foetal specimen under 8 weeks of life. Anatomical relationship among skeletal structures (still cartilaginous) invites to understand that transitional anomalies may be likely to occur. (*Cl* clivus, *Od* odontoid process, *At* Anterior arc of the atlas, *Ax* vertebral body of the axis, *C3* Vertebral body of C3, *SC* Spinal cord)

de tip of a well formed odontoid process (Fig. 14.5). Ossification anomalies of the independent nuclei of the apical and central portions may lead to abnormal formation of the odontoid which would ossify independently leading to the os odontoideum anomaly [4, 22–26].

Variations of the time of normal ossification in the odontoid itself, between 4 and 18 years of age, may lead to different morphologies of the odontoid process which may show some fibrous or cartilaginous remnant between the odontoid and the vertebral body of C2 in almost one-third of normal adults [23].

14.3 Congenital Malformations of the Odontoid Process

The anomalies of the odontoid process are currently total or partial defects of formation, sometimes associated with fusion to the upper portion of the odontoid with the anterior arch of the atlas or one of its articular processes. As in many conditions that may be asymptomatic their frequency is unknown but more common than appreciated. These anomalies are usually discovered in patients undergoing radiological studies following a trauma to the neck. The most frequent are the following: Ossiculum terminale, os odontoideum, aplasia or hypoplasia of the odontoid, biphid or duplicated odontoid and hyperplasia [15, 22–24, 27–29].

Although the distinction of aplasia or hypoplasia from os odontoideum is only radiographic and of limited importance, they all will be described separately. Nevertheless, the only relevant thing is the C1–C2 instability and its clinical repercussion.

14.3.1 Ossiculum Terminale

Anomalies of the cranial tip of the odontoid are the rarest of this group. This morphologic anomaly involves a failure of fusion of the apical segment of the dens with the basal portions or it is otherwise originated as a remnant of the notochorde, included in the terminal or apical ligament which connects the odontoid process and the basilar lamina. Ossiculum terminale is currently observed as a small rounded piece of bone and, normally, it has not clinical relevance due to the lack of repercussion. It has to be differentiated from the so called "third condyle", a small bone included in the apical ligament very close to the foramen magnum. It may be considered as a representative of the body of an occipital vertebra or a proatlas [2, 22, 24, 29–31].

Ossiculum terminale is normally a non relevant finding which has no clinical repercussion although some authors have reported ossiculum terminale with cervical cord compression and atlantoaxial dislocation, quadriplegia and death [22]. Except for this exceptional possibility, the only problem may arise in the difficulty to differentiate ossiculum terminale from os odontoideum or a traumatic lesion. This possible mistake may be solved by making a dynamic radiographic study to confirm normal stability.

14.3.2 Os Odontoideum

This anomaly is also called congenital pseudoarthrosis and comes from a failure of fusion of the odontoid and the arch centers; it is the most frequent and important congenital malformation of the axis, the prototype of congenital anomaly leading to segmental instability [7, 24]. It was first described by Giacomini in 1886 in a female with cretinism by post-mortem examination. There was an abnormal joint-like articulation separating the os odontoideum from the body of the axis [22].

In this anomaly, the odontoid usually develops to normal proportions but union with the body of the axis is deficient. The upper part of the odontoid appears as a rounded bone which maintains its normal relations to the anterior arch and the articular processes of the atlas but is more or less separated from the body of the axis and a more or less evident bony prominence of the remnant lower part of the odontoid on the upper side of the vertebral body.

Most of times, os odontoideum may be located in a high position at the normal place of the tip of the dens (orthotopic), having always a wide space of separation from its remnant at the base (if any), and it may be also placed near the basal occiput (Dystopic) where it may be fused to the clivus. The os odontoideum may be also fused to the anterior arch or an articular process of the atlas.

The anomaly may be present throughout life with no symptoms but it may produce symptoms progressively or come to light following a cervico-occipital trauma. Nuchal or high neck discomfort or pain are common and may be associated with a variety of neurological symptoms—even tetraparesis or transient paralysis—due to cord compression between the upper-posterior part of the vertebral body and the posterior arch of the atlas and repeated micro-trauma with normal neck movements.

Concerning the origin of the os odontoideum, despite it seems to be clearly explained and understood from an embryological point of view, there is not always agreement about its congenital origin and there are arguments in favour of a traumatic origin: (1) Frequent antecedent of an ancient trauma; (2) Rare association with other congenital anomalies; (3) Lack of accurate embryologic explanation; (4) Report of cases of documented normal odontoid process which evolved to os odontoideum after a trauma [3–22]. The cartilaginous epiphyseal plate would prevent revascularization contributing to resorption of bone and non-union, an "acquired" os odontoideum. Infection has been also related as an acquired cause of os odontoideum [32].

The recommended radiological studies are lateral neutral and flexion–extension views and open mouth neutral and dynamic left and right inclination views. Lateral roentgenograms currently allow to detect the abnormality and dynamic studies demonstrate the hypermobility in both sagittal (flexion and extension lateral views) and coronal planes (lateral inclination in transoral views) (Fig. 14.6). The atlas may appear subluxated or dislocated on the axis (usually forwards) with the dynamic studies or even in neutral position. When subluxation or dislocation is detected in neutral position, dynamic studies to quantify the instability have to be performed.

Some confusion may exist when facing an image in which a thin radio-transparent line is observed at the base of the odontoid in a patient younger than 12. In such a case, a dynamic radiological study is mandatory to distinguish a remnant of cartilage separating the body and the dens from a fracture line or an os odontoideum. Mistakes may also exist in case of a real fracture of the dens base or traumatic dens separation, similar to an epiphyseal detachment (Fig. 14.7). Os odontoideum is a corticated round or oval ossicle of about 1 cm separated from the base of the odontoid by a variable gap. Its radiological appearance may vary either in size and shape as well as in bony density or thickness of the "cortical" contour (Fig. 14.8). Frequently, the anterior arch of the atlas appears to be hypertrophic, more dense and having the "cortical" thicker than normal. Fusion to the clivus, anterior arch of the atlas or an articular process are not usually seen in standard radiographs but they are perfectly determined with CT scan views (Fig. 14.9). Old ununited dens fractures may be hard to differentiate from the congenital malformation. CT or MRI may also help to better observe, define and understand the possible neurological repercussion of the instability on

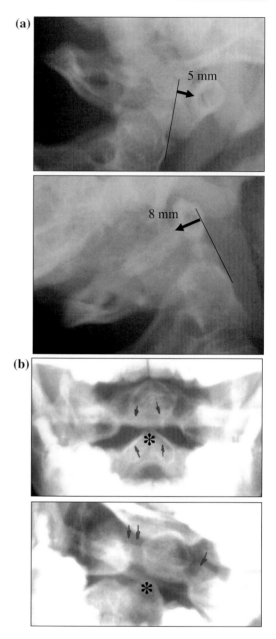

Fig. 14.6 **a** Lateral dynamic radiograph shows C1–C2 hypermobility (13 mm) in the sagittal plane. **b** Transoral dynamic radiograph shows a neutral position (*above*) and lateral displacement to the *left side* (*below*) (with permission of the Spanish journal of Orthopaedic Surgery and Traumatology, Rev Ortop Traum, Ref. [34]). *Above* The small remnant at the base of the odontoid (*star*) is well aligned with the os odontoideum in neutral position (*small arrows*). *Below* The os odontoideum moves laterally with the inclination of the head changing relationship with the remnant base (*star*). Fusion between os odontoideum and articular processes of the atlas seems to be defined (*small arrows*)

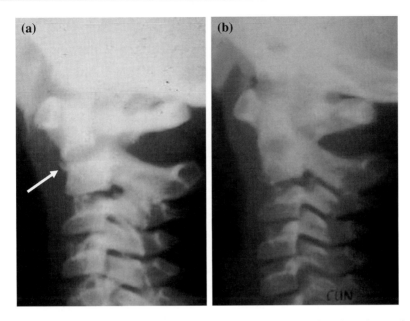

Fig. 14.7 **a** A 9-year-old boy with a misdiagnosed synchondrosis at the base of the odontoid process, after being run over by a motorcycle. One month later on consulted with persistent suboccipital pain. Our diagnose was fracture at the base of the odontoid, slightly displaced (look at the posterior alignment of the odontoid and C2 body) and possibly through a persistent synchondrosis with a small bony fragment detached from the body (*arrow*). This case dates before the era of axial imaging (CT and MRI), **b** Bone healing of the fracture after 6 weeks of immobilization in a SOMI brace

the spinal cord (alterations of the cord contour or signal alterations compatible with myelomalacia) (Fig. 14.10).

The normal consequence of this anomaly is a more or less intense atlantoaxial instability because of forward slippage of C1 on C2 (mainly), but also due to abnormal lateral displacement of C1 on C2. During normal movement, os odontoideum remains fixed to the anterior arch of the atlas by the transverse ligaments. Symptoms appear by abnormal mobility in C1–C2 joints and by spinal cord impingement between (mainly) the posterior arch of the atlas and the basal rudiment of the dens attached to the body of C2.

The most common symptoms—if any—of the resulting instability are: posterior head ache, suboccipital pain, vague neck discomfort, torticollis or stiff neck due to defensive spasm, transient stroke after neck rotation (in adults), variable degree of extremities weakness and/or sensory defects or numbness, clonus, sphincter disturbances and spastic tetraparesis. A small number of patients may have symptoms and signs of cerebral and brain stem ischemia, seizures, syncope, vertigo, visual disturbances and mental deterioration. These alterations have been related with vertebral artery compression at the foramen magnum or just below it. In cases with these symptoms, a careful neurological differential diagnosis is mandatory [32, 33]. Neurological symptoms have been reported as existing in 45 % of the patients or more [32, 34, 35]. These symptoms may appear in a slowly progressive way or abruptly, as an acute expression of the effect of a head or neck trauma. Congenital anomalies diagnosed in children or adolescents are more likely to occur without neurological lesion than those diagnosed in adults.

Whatever may be the way of arriving to an accurate diagnosis, even with no symptoms or a poorly expressive clinical picture, once the doctor realize that the patient has an os

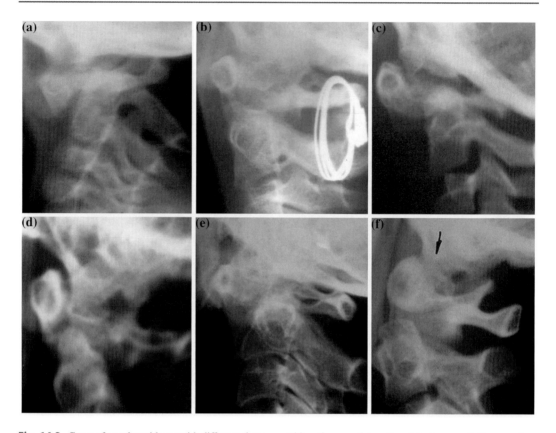

Fig. 14.8 Cases of os odontoideum with different shape, dimensions, separation from the base, bone density and corticalization. Shape, dimension and corticalization of the anterior arch of the atlas are also diverse. Cases **a**, **b** and **c** show variable degrees of anterior C1−C2 subluxation or dislocation (**a**). In case **f**, the os odontoideum is fused to the anterior arch of the atlas (Same case that Fig. 14.9a). Figure **a**, **b**, **c** and **f**, with permission of the Spanish Journal of Orthopaedic Surgery and Traumatology, Rev Ortop Traum, Ref. [34]

odontoideum and objective signs of instability, the patient has to be informed on the risks of having progressive neurological impairment or a tragic, catastrophic consequences in case of accident. When the patient is a child, even asymptomatic, parents are frequently stroked by understanding the amount of normal activities in the daily life which are a real danger for their child. Therefore, either adults as well as young patients should not be treated conservatively and the current therapeutic indication is surgical treatment with C1−C2 fusion [36]. In some special case—as in patients with Down' syndrome having also occipitocervical instability—fusion may be extended to the occiput.

14.3.3 Aplasia or Hypoplasia (Complete or Partial Absence) of the Odontoid

Aplasia of the odontoid process is particularly rare. Trauma and infection have also reported as acquired causes of hypoplastic odontoid process [7, 32]. It is easy to detect in transoral radiological exams and leads usually to a more or less pronounced C1−C2 instability. Surgical treatment with C1−C2 posterior fusion is usually indicated. We may include here the agenesis of the vertebral body—partial or total—which is always accompanied by absence of the odontoid process and implies precocious and severe

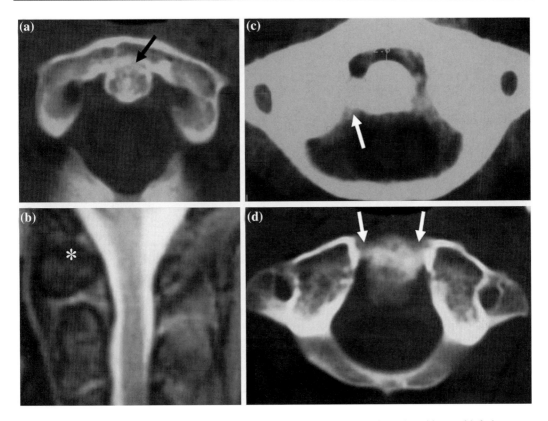

Fig. 14.9 a and **b** Axial and sagittal views of os odontoideum fused to the anterior arch of the atlas (*black arrow* in **a**, and *star* in **b** on the *upper part* of an imaginary line which should separate between anterior arch of the atlas and os odontoideum). **c** and **d** Axial views of two cases of os odontoideum with fusion to one (**c**, *arrow*) or two articular processes (**d**, *arrows*), (Figures a and c, with permission of the Spanish Journal of Orthopaedic Surgery and Traumatology, Rev Ortop Traum, Ref. [34])

neurological alterations due to instability and spinal cord compression. When the odontoid is absent, a slight depression between the upper articular processes may be seen in the open mouth view. In contrast with the os odontoideum anomaly, many patients with agenesis of the dens have significant posterior subluxation [32].

Hypoplasia is more common. A rudimentary odontoid, hypoplastic, abnormally small or absent, may favour atlantoaxial instability. As previously mentioned, the only distinctive features being radiographic, separating aplasia or hypoplasia from os odontoideum is of limited importance

since they usually lead to instability and similar symptoms, signs and treatment are identical.

Neurological alterations and objective signs of instability would make surgical stabilization advisable.

14.3.4 Biphid or Duplicated Ododontoid

Some delay in the normal ossification of the secondary nucleus of the tip of the odontoid or variations in its normal development, may lead to a

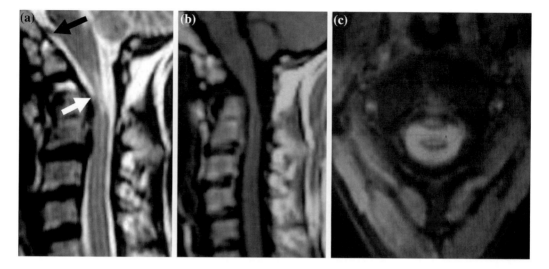

Fig. 14.10 **a** and **b** T2 (**a**) and T1 (**b**) weighted sagittal views of a 42-year-old patient affected of Down's syndrome, having C1–C2 hypermobility and tetraparesis. Thinness of the spinal cord and changes of myelomalatia are evident behind the body of C2 (*white arrow*). Some degree of fusion seems to exist between os odontoideum, clivus and anterior arch of the atlas (*black arrow*). **c** Axial view in which is also evident the thinness of the spinal cord at the zone of compression due to instability. (Figure c, with permission of the Spanish Journal of Orthopaedic Surgery and Traumatology, Rev Ortop Traum, Ref. [34])

biphid radiological look of the tip of a quite normal odontoid. More or les frequently, at the end of growth, this secondary nucleus remains as non-fused ossicle, similar to the ossiculum terminale. In these cases, usually, there is not instability or other clinical repercussion [7, 37–39].

Duplicated odontoid is very rare and the embryologic anomaly responsible of its occurrence is unknown but it is more likely to occur as result of the lack of fusion of the two primary centres appearing normally at about the fifth-sixth month of fetal life on each side of the midline.

A transoral view of a standard radiograph is usually enough to appreciate the duplication of the dens and CT with multiplanar reformatting allows assessing this anomaly completely. Association with other malformations as fusion of the anterior lip of the foramen magnum and the anterior arch of C1, midline assicles on this anterior arch, bipartite atlas or os odontoideum have been described.

Clinical symptoms may vary from suboccipital painful complaints to reduction of the ability to rotate the neck to tetraplegia after a trauma in a young patient aged 13 who associated os odontoideum and a synovial cyst [28].

Surgical treatment may be indicated in case of instability or spinal cord compression. In the above mentioned case by Weng et al. [28], decompression was obtained by reduction of C1–C2 subluxation and stabilization was achieved by O–C2 instrumented fusion, the patient being totally recovered from the neurological point of view.

14.3.5 Hyperplasia of the Odontoid

It is very rarely observed as an isolated malformation. The dens exceeds vertically its relationship with the anterior arch of the atlas and may contact with the clivus and cross the Chamberlain's line (Fig. 14.11). Currently it not represents a clinical problem unless it would exits an associated C1–C2 instability. In such a case, the exceeding apical part of the dens would be a traumatic agent producing cord compression or a cord injury in case of accident [22].

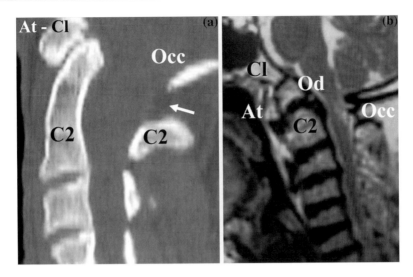

Fig. 14.11 a Sagittal CT scan of the cervical spine shows hyperplasia of the odontoid process (*At-Cl Atlas-Clivus, Occ Occipital bone, C2 axis, White arrow* absence of the posterior arch of the atlas). **b** T2 weighted MRI sagittal view of a congenitally abnormal occipito-cervical junction in which the tip of the odontoid process (which is not yet fused with the vertebral body) is contacting the clivus by means of an apparent synchondrosis. The image belong to a 8-year-old boy with spondylo-epiphyseal dysplasia. (*Cl* clivus, *Od* odontoid process, *At* anterior arch of the atlas, *C2* vertebral body of the axis, *Occ* occipital bone)

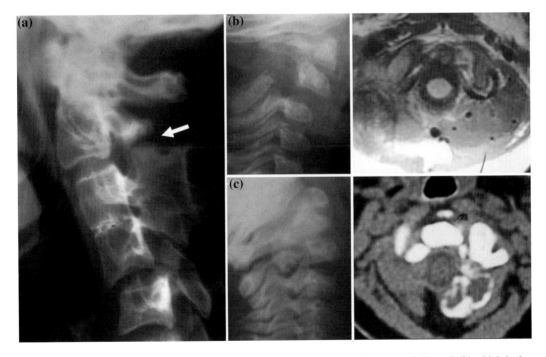

Fig. 14.12 a. Lateral view of a congenital spondylolysis (*arrow*) with C2–C3 congenital block and instability at C4–C5 level (with permission of the Spanish journal of paediatrics, Acta Pediátr Esp, Ref. [40]). **b** and **c** Evident defect of the pars interticularis-pedicle of the axis in a 4-month-old child with lysthesis. Pathological evaluation reported a "pseudo-tumor calcificans" (**b**) which had an spontaneous ossification and reconstruction (**c**). It would be an obstetric trauma with fracture of the isthmus and a dystrophic bone healing (with permission of the Spanish journal of paediatrics, Acta Pediátr Esp, Ref. [40])

14.4 Congenital Malformations of the Isthmus/Pedicle

The most frequent anomaly observed at the level of the pars interarticularis or the pedicle of C2 are the existence of a cartilaginous remnant or an evident pseudoarthrosis (Fig. 14.12), sometimes with spondylolisthesis. Isthmic/pedicular defects are frequently associated with spina bifida. Although congenital spondylolisthesis is generally reported at the sixth cervical (24) vertebra it may be also observed more or less frequently at C4, C5 and C7 levels and very rarely at C2 level. So rarely that is a real paucity of literature to consult [1–3, 23, 24, 40–44].

A part from the possible difficulties of recognizing the anomalies, their repercussion is not important and reports of evident instability and/or symptomatic patients are exceptional. Some problems may exist in case of image studies after trauma, being difficult to distinguish congenital pseudoarthrosis from a fracture [40–43]. The present options of image studies grant normally the differential diagnosis.

Arriola et al. [40] report the cases of three patients (aged 9 months and 19 and 33 years) presenting with neck pain (two patients) and torticollis (one patient). Radiological studies gave the diagnosis: isthmic spondylolysis without instability in the two patients aged 19 and 33; the child aged 9 months did not have any traumatic antecedent and had spondylolysis of C2 with apparent C2–C3 subluxation and a calcified mass around the left pedicle/isthmus. This patient was operated on in other hospital and the report of the biopsy concluded that the condition was tumoral calcinosis. After intralesional resection of the calcified mass the isthmic defect disappear in both sides, total bony union being observed at the age of 2. We thought that some isthmic defect was present at birth and some obstetric local trauma provoked a haematoma and the pathological alteration which finally lead to the healing of the defect. Differential diagnosis with a fracture was impossible.

Agenesis of the pedicles is very rare as isolated anomaly and it may be observed in case of a more complex malformation or in a poli-malformative syndrome [44]. In case of objective instability, with hypermobility between C2 and C3, chronic painful complaints or myelopathy, C2–C3 fusion is indicated (Fig. 14.13).

14.5 Congenital Malformations of the Lamina and Spinous Process

Laminae may be involved in a malformation appearing with lack of formation of the posterior arch, as a wide spina bifida with lack the spinous process and a more or less open window between left and right sides of the posterior arch depending on the degree of agenesis of the laminae, which may be total and sometimes involved in an unstable malformation if it is a part of a complete aplasia of the posterior arch of C2, thus including the articular processes.

On the other hand, laminae and spinous process may be fused to its correspondent at C3 level and more rarely to the posterior arch of the atlas (Fig. 14.14).

In daily practice, partial absence of the posterior arch due to lack of formation or normal union of laminae and spinous process may be a problem only in case of an operation by posterior approach. If the posterior arch "window" is neglected, surgeon may enter the canal with instruments and injure the dura and the spinal cord.

14.6 Synostoses or Congenital Fusions

The clinical significance of a defect of segmentation is related to the influence that the "block" may have on the development of instability or degeneration at the adjacent segments. Congenital anomalies may come mainly from defects of differentiation between the occiput and C1 and defects of differentiation between C2 and C3 [2, 11, 38, 45, 46].

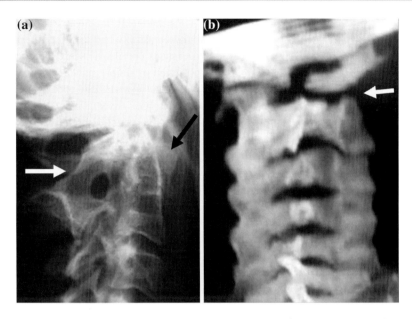

Fig. 14.13 a Oblique radiograph of the upper cervical spine with partial agenesis of the lower part of an articular process of C1 (which appears tilted on C2, *black arrow*) and agenesis a pedicle and the upper part of an articular process of C2, appearing the opposite one with single contour overlapped with the posterior arch of the atlas (*white arrow*). **b** Frontal view of a tridimensional reconstruction of the same case, showing the bony defect (*arrow*) due to the agenesis of the lower part of the right articular process of C1, its corresponding articular process at C2 and the right pedicle. The caudal aspect of the pars interarticularis and the lower articular process of C2 remain

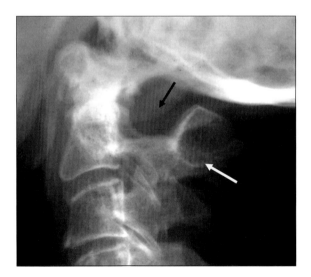

Fig. 14.14 Lateral radiograph shows fusion of the posterior arches of C1 and C2 (*white arrow*). Note that there is a lack of continuity in the lateral junction between the articular processes of the atlas and its posterior arch (*black arrow*) which as been defined as lateral spina bifida of the atlas [19]

14.6.1 *Fusion*

This is the most commonly recognized occipitocervical anomaly and it is characterized by partial or total complete fusion of the bony ring of the atlas to the occiput. It is called occipitalization or assimilation of the atlas and may occur as a consequence of a defect in the development of the caudal half of the last occipital sclerotome and the cranial half of the first cervical sclerotome. The lack of flexion–extension mobility at O–C1 level may determine progressive laxity of the transverse ligament and hypermobility between atlas and axis leading to local symptoms and indeterminacy on a potential risk of cord compression. Twenty percent of the patients have associated other cranial, facial or vertebral bony malformation [2, 30].

Symptoms are characteristics of those conditions with instability at the upper cervical spine, the patients being frequently asymptomatic or complaining of suboccipital pain, painful muscle spasm, torticollis and/or a wide diversity of neurological signs and symptoms of cord compression. The onset of symptoms is usually at third or fourth decade, being the beginning insidious. Although progression of symptoms is usually slow sudden aggravation and instant death have been reported even without a trauma [47, 48]. Local swelling from infection of the nasopharynx or pharynx may initiate symptoms and complaints. When symptoms have a sudden onset in adults without a precipitating cause differential diagnosis must include multiple sclerosis or amyotrophic lateral sclerosis.

Late onset of symptoms would be reasonably due to gradual laxity of C1–C2 ligaments—notably the transverse one—provoking intermittent narrowing of the spinal canal between the posterior part of the tip of the dens and the posterior arch of the atlas. Spinal cord compression is greater when the odontoid process is relatively high respecting to the anterior arch of the atlas (it may then enter in the foramen magnum) and in the case of synostosis of C2–C3 or longer.

Radiological diagnosis is not difficult. When bony continuity between the ring of C1 and the occiput is not clearly seen, there are some sings observed in simple standard radiographic lateral views that usually lead to suspect that atlas and occiput are fused. This signs are: Basilar impression, which is "relative" when the ring of C1 is very thin, less high than normal; very high position of C1, appearing too close to the occiput; and very high position of the anterior arch of C1 respecting to the dens, appearing quite at its tip. The odontoid often has an abnormal shape, is longer than normal and its angle with the base of the axis is directed more posteriorly.

Anyway, in case of suspicion, 3D multiplanar CT allows to an easy demonstration of the union between the occiput and C1, specially in coronal and sagittal reconstructions [12]. In the very young population, image interpretation and radiologic diagnosis may be frequently difficult because a variable but sometimes significant portion of the ring of C1 is unossified.

Atlantoaxial interval has not to be greater than 4–5 mm in dynamic radiological lateral view studies. If real instability is detected, explanation on the potential risk in case of progressive instability or accident has to be given to the patient and OC2 fusion may be advised and periodical review has to be recommended. Cord compression is more frequent in case of narrow canal between the tip of the odontoid and the posterior lip of the foramen magnum.

Isolated congenital C1–C2 hypermobility with no bony anomalies may be observed in some cases, more frequently in people with Down syndrome [13, 30]. The cause would be a congenitally determined laxity or absence of the transverse ligament.

Fusion or defect of segmentation from the occiput may also include more cervical vertebrae as the axis and others more caudal, within the group of variants which we may observe and classify more or less correctly as Klippel-Feil syndrome. Vertebral congenital blocks may exist with no brevicollis or low posterior hairline.

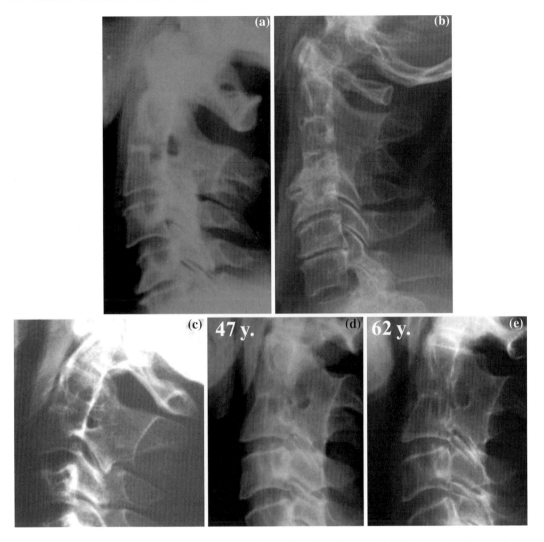

Fig. 14.15 a A 55-year-old patient with a C2−C3 congenital block and no degenerative changes at the adjacent level and evident degeneration at levels C4−C5 (listhesis) and C5−C6 (osteophytes, diminished discal high). **b** Patient aged 50 with a C2−C4 congenital block and advanced C4−C7 degeneration. **c** Patient aged 48 with a C2−C3 congenital block and no adjacent degeneration. **d** and **e** Patient with a C2−C3 congenital block consulting twice for pain on the cervico-thoracic junction at the ages of 47 (**d**) and 62 (**e**). No degeneration was observed at the adjacent levels

When progressive hypermobility is demonstrated or patients become symptomatic surgical treatment has to be considered. Some times a conservative trial with traction or immobilization with collar or SOMI brace, may be adequate when symptoms appear after a trauma. Posterior O−C2 fusion is the normal surgical indication, sometimes associated to resection of the posterior arch of C1 and suboccipital craniectomy depending on the neurological deficit.

14.6.2 Atlanto-Axial Fusion

Although we have some times observed partial synostoses connecting Atlas and Axis, even persistent synchondrosis between occiput and the tip of the odontoid process (Fig. 14.11) complete atlanto-axial congenital fusion is exceptionally reported out of the possible fusions to the arch or the articular process of C1 seen in case of os odontoideum [2, 3].

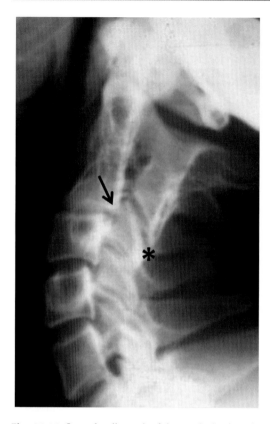

Fig. 14.16 Lateral radiograph of the cervical spine of a 48-year-old woman who felt a transient tetraparesis after a fall while skiing. She had a frontal impact and the subsequent abrupt hyper-extension of the neck being quite tetraplegic for 5 min. The radiograph sowed congenital stenosis (lines at the base of the spinous process close or contacting the posterior line of the articular process) and retrolisthesis of the C2C3 block on C4. The postero-inferior border of C3 being displaced posteriorly and entering the canal (arrow) with separation of the articular process of C4 and C5 (*star*)

14.6.3 C2−C3 fusion

Together with congenital synostosis at C4−C5 or C5−C6 levels, this defect of segmentation is quite common either as isolated finding as well as a part in a more extended block in a Klippel-Feil syndrome. In the classic Klippel-Feil syndrome, the neck is short and the posterior hair line appears very low. Some authors consider that cervical blocks cause degeneration of the adjacent segments [49, 50] but others think that it is considered to be even an incidental finding [51] unrelated to disease, specially at C2−C3

level. We think that it depends on the number of mobile segments involved in the congenital synostosis and also on the position in the cervical spine, degeneration being very common in the levels in which degeneration is common— C5 to C7—and is more rare at C3−C4 level in case of C2−C3 congenital synostosis. Although C2−C3 congenital fusion may be associated to degeneration at C3−C4 level, of course, it would be generally benign [7] and very well tolerated; in our daily practice we frequently observe patients older than fifty or sixty who complaint of low cervical pain with a well corresponding degeneration at C5−C7 levels and a congenital C2−C3 block with no degeneration at all at C3−C4 level (Fig. 14.15).

People with a C2−C3 block may be asymptomatic all along their life but sometimes patients complain of middle neck pain or stiffness because of adjacent degeneration, specially in cases of fusion at several segments. Furthermore, there are reports on cases of C2−C3 congenital blocks having myelopathy (even in an eighteen-year-old boy [45]) or transient tetraparesis [52] in case of minor trauma with no fracture or dislocation. In these cases, the association of a small hypermobility/instability and a narrow canal is currently the cause of a neural lesion (Fig. 14.16).

Radiological diagnosis is usually easy, either as a part of a Klippel-Feil syndrome as well as in the case of a localized block, limited at C2−C3 level. The shape of the vertebral bodies is usually normal or minimally distorted, the articular processes and the laminae appear totally fused, the spinous process being frequently partially fused. The disc remnant is more or less visible but easily recognized. Coming back on adjacent degeneration, Moon et al. [11] reported that normally aligned congenital synostosis of C2−C3 is rarely associated with a junctional problem, whereas a kyphotic synostosis is associated with a caudal junctional problem. They also conclude that cervical spondylosis developing after the age of 40 is not associated with C2−C3 synostosis.

Cases with multiple level synostosis (frequently associated with segmental stenosis, at the block levels and transitional zones) are more

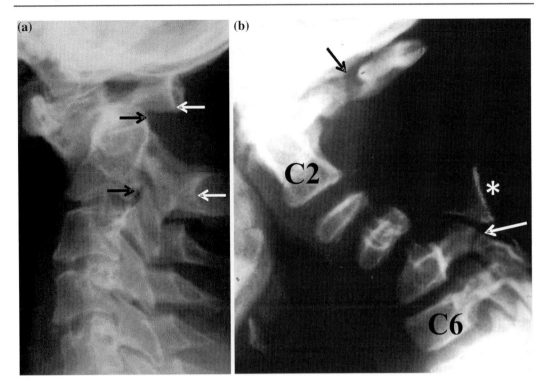

Fig. 14.17 a Lateral radiograph of the cervical spine of a 42-year-old man with Down's syndrome and os odontoideum and evident C1–C2 instability correlating with a clinical picture of spastic tetraparesis. He is the same patient than the one of Fig. 14.10, were appeared with a better alignment due to the supine position required for MRI studies. Instability lead to compression at C1–C2 level (*upper arrows*). Dimensions of the canal at this point may be compared with the ones at C2–C3 level (*lower arrows*). This is the paradigm of a congenital anomaly of the axis leading to indication for arthrodesis. **b.** Lateral radiograph of the cervical spine of an 8-year-old girl showing a very complex congenital anomaly with no discussion on a possible instability and its subsequent indication for arthrodesis. There is a total absence of posterior structures of C2 to C4, except a small reminder of articular process and lamina of C4 (*star*), defect of formation of the body of C5, spondylolysis of C5 (*white arrow*), assimilation of the atlas and lateral spina bifida [18, 19] (*black arrow*)

prone to have neurological symptoms. Congenital synostosis present sometime problems in the differential diagnosis but image studies and genetics lead easily to an accurate diagnosis [46].

Treatment depends on the clinical picture and may be conservative in absence of neurological symptoms, or surgical in case of persistent pain or neurological signs. Surgical treatment generally consists of fusion of the adjacent degenerated segments, associated or not to cord decompression. Yi et al. [17] have reported surgical management of the adjacent degenerated segment with total disc replacement; it appears to be promising but we need studies on series and long-term outcome to feel sure on the indications and the possible "survival" of a prosthetic mobile segment under a more or less long vertebral synostosis.

14.7 Mixed Congenital Malformations

Association anomalies may cause very complex malformations, difficult to define and distinguish due to combination of agenesis of parts of a vertebral ring and partial or total fusion among several vertebral units. These mixed malformations often involve more than four vertebrae and are a part of a polymalformative syndrome [28, 53]. The most common mixed anomalies are not very complex and have been already mentioned, the association of assimilation of the atlas to a block between C2 and C3, and the association between os odontoideum and spina bifida of the atlas.

A part of the more or less accurate definition of the type of anomalies being a part of the mixed and more complex one, from a practical point of view, surgeon try to determine if there is instability and its potential repercussion in terms of future neurological risk or correlation (Fig. 14.17).

References

1. Bailey RW, Sherk HH, Dunn EJ et al (eds) (1983) The cervical spine. The Cervical Spine Research Society, Lippincott, London
2. Epstein BS (1964) The spine. A radiological text and atlas. Lea & Febiger, Philadelphia
3. Roy-Camille R, Doursounian L, Henry P et al (1986) Les malformations osseuses de la Charnière Cranio-Rachidienne. In: Roy-Camille R (ed) Rachis Cervical Supérieur. Cinquièmes Journées d'Orthopédie de la Pitié, Masson, Paris, pp 3–10
4. Roy-Camille R, Léonard Ph, Mamoudy P (1986) Embriologie et Phylogenèse. de l'Articulation Cranio-vertébrale. In: Roy-Camille R (ed) Rachis cervical Supérieur. Cinquièmes Journées d'Orthopédie de la Pitié, Masson, Paris, pp 3–10
5. Sherk HH, Fielding JW (eds) (1978) Symposium on the upper cervical spine. Orthop Clin North Am 9(4): 865–1143
6. Mallet JF, Lechevallier J (eds) (1993) Chirurgie et Orthopédie du Rachis Cervical de l'enfant. Monographie du Group d'Étude en Orthopédie Pédiatrique. Sauramps Médical, Montpellier
7. Touzet PH (1993) Les malformations vertébrales du rachis cervical. In: Mallet JF, Lechevallier J (eds) Chirurgie et Orthopédie du Rachis Cervical de l'enfant. Monographie du Group d'Étude en Orthopédie Pédiatrique. Sauramps Médical, Montpellier, pp 101–114
8. Shapiro R, Youngberg AS, Rothman SLG (1973) The differential diagnosis of traumatic lesions of the occipito-atlanto-axial segment. Radiol Clin North Amer XI:505–526
9. Ding X, Abumi K, Ito M et al (2012) A retrospective study of congenital osseous anomalies at the craniocervictreated by occipitocervical plate-rod system. Eur Spine J 21:1580–1589
10. Holmes JC, Hall J (1978) Fusion for instability and potential instability of the cervical spine in children and adolescents. In: Sherk HH, Fielding JW (eds) The upper cervical spine. Orthop Clin North Amer Vol 9/4. Saunders, Philadelpuia, pp 923–943
11. Moon MS, Kim SS, Lee BJ et al (2010) Radiographic assessment of congenital C2–C3 synostosis. J Orthop Surg 18:143–147
12. Newton PO, Hahn GW, Fricka KB et al (2002) Utility of three-dimensional and multiplanar reformatted computed tomography for evaluation of pedriatric congenital spine abnormalities. Spine 27:844–850
13. Garbayo AJ, Villas C (1988) Luxación atlas-axis en el síndrome de Down. Rev Ortop Traum 32IB:213–217
14. Leyes M, Martínez-Peric R, Amillo S et al (1994) Displasia de dygge-melchior-clausen: consideraciones diagnósticas y tratamiento ortopédico. Acta Pediátr Esp 52:100–104
15. Li XF, Jiang WM, Yang HL et al (2011) Surgical treatment of chronic C1–C2 dislocation with absence od odontoid process using C1 hooks with C2 pedicle screws. Spine 36:E1245–E1249
16. Reilly CW, Choit RL (2006) Transarticular screws in the management of C1–C2 instability in children. J Pediatr Orthop 26:582–588
17. Yi S, Kim SH, Shin HC et al (2007) Cervical arthroplasty in a patient with Klippel-Feil syndrome. Acta Neurochir 149:805–809
18. Villas C (1994) Malformations congénitales de l'atlas. Rev Chir Orthop 80:162
19. Villas C, Vides RE, Yáñez R (1990) Malformaciones congénitas del atlas. Clasificación y repercusión clínica. Rev Med Univ Navarra 34:157–162
20. Villas C, Alfonso M, Romero LM et al (2010) Long-term outcome of children undergoing Brooks-Jenkins' technique for atlanto-axial instability or dislocation. Eur Spine J 19:1061
21. Alfonso M, Villas C, Romero LM et al (2010) C1–C2 luxation in children with down syndrome: long term evolution of two patients treated with C1–C2 fusion. Eur Spine J 19:179
22. Truex RC, Johnson CH (1978) Congenital abnormalities of the upper cervical spine. In: Sherk HH, Fielding JW (eds) The upper cervical spine. Orthop Clin North Amer Vol 9/4. Saunders, Philadelpuia, pp 891–900
23. Sherk HH, Parke WW (1983) Developmental anatomy. In: Bailey RW, Sherk HH, Dunn EJ et al (eds) The cervical spine. Chapter 1: anatomy, The Cervical Spine Research Society, Lippincott, London, pp 1–8
24. Bateman JE (1978) Evolution, embryology, and congenital anomalies. In: The shoulder and neck: chapter 1, Saunders, Philadelphia, pp 1–46
25. Crockard HA, Stevens JM (1995) Craniovertebral junction anomalies in inherited disorders: part of the syndrome or caused by the disorder? Eur J Pediatr 154:504–512
26. Stevens JM, Chong WK, Barber C et al (1994) A new appraisal of abnormalities of the odontoid process associated with atlanto-axial subluxation and neurological disability. Brain 117:133–148

27. Arvin B, Fournier-Gosselin MP, Fehlings MG (2010) Os odontoideum: etiology and surgical management. Neurosurgery 66:A22–A31

28. Weng C, Wang LM, Wang WD et al (2010) Bipartite atlas with os odontoideum and synovial cyst. Spine 35:E568–E575

29. Sherk HH, Nicholson J (1969) Rotatory atlanto-axial dislocation associated with ossiculum terminale and mongolism. J Bone Joint Surg 51A:957–964

30. Hensinger RN (1983) Congenital anomalies of the atlantoaxial joint. In: Bailey RW, Sherk HH, Dunn EJ et al (eds) The cervical spine. Chapter 5: congenital malformations, The cervical Spine Research Society, Lippincott, London, pp 155–160

31. Hensinger RN (1983) Congenital anomalies of the odontoid. In: Bailey RW, Sherk HH, Dunn EJ et al (eds) The cervical spine. Chapter 5: congenital malformations, The Cervical Spine Research Society, Lippincott, London, pp 164–174

32. Hensinger RN, Fielding J, Hawkins RJ (1978) Congenital anomalies of the odontoid process. In: Sherk HH, Fielding JW (eds) The upper cervical spine. Orthop Clin North Amer Vol 9/4. Saunders, Philadelpuia, pp 901–912

33. Rowland LP, Shapiro JH, Jacobson HG (1958) Neurological syndromes associated with congenital absence of the odontoid process. Arch Neurol Psychiat 60:286–291

34. Villas C, Arriola F, Vital JM et al (2001) Tratamiento del os odontoideum. Revisión de 18 casos. Rev Ortop Traum 45 (Suppl 1):37–47

35. Villas C, Vital JM, Denaro E (2001) Treatment of os odontoideum: a multicentric study. Eur Spine J 10(Suppl 1):44

36. Arriola FJ, Mora G, Villas C (1995) Tratamiento quirúrgico de las anomalias tipo os-odontoideum: a propósito de 7 casos. In: Columna vertebral, Fundación Mapfre Medicina, Madrid, pp 183–197

37. Garant M, Oudjhanc K, Sinsky A et al (1997) Duplicated odontoid process: plain radiographic and CT appearance of a rare congenital anomaly of the cervical spine. AJNR 18:1719–1720

38. Dilettoso S, Uccello M, Dilettoso A et al (2012) Duplicated odontoid process and atlas clefts associated to Klippel-Feil syndrome. Spine J 12: 449–450

39. Osti M, Philipp H, Meusburger B et al (2006) Os odontoideum with bipartite atlas and segmental instability: case report. Eur Spine J 15(Suppl 5):564–567

40. Arriola FJ, Villas C, Mora G (1998) Espondilolisis primaria del axis. a propósito de tres casos. Acta Pediátr Esp 56:53–57

41. Hasue M, Kikuchi S, Matsui T et al (1983) Spondylolysis of the axis. Report of four cases. Spine 8:901–906

42. Matthews LS, Vetter WL, Tolo VT (1982) Cervical anomaly simulating hangman's fracture in a child. Case report. J Bone Joint Surg 64A:299–300

43. Smith JT, Skinner SR, Shonnard NH (1993) Persistent synchondrosis of the second cervical vertebra simulating a hangman's fracture in a child. J Bone Joint Surg 75A:1228–1230

44. Currarino G (1989) Primary spondylolisthesis of the axis vertebra (C2) in three children, including one with pyknodisostosis. Pediatr Radiol 19:535–538

45. Epstein NE, Epstein JA, Zilkha A (1984) Traumatic myelopathy in a seventeen-year old child with cervical spinal stenosis (without fracture or dislocation) and a C2–C3 Klippel-Feil fusion. A case report. Spine 9:344–347

46. Schaffer AA, Kaplan FS, Tracy MR et al (2005) Developmental anomalies of the cervical spine in patients with fibrodysplasia ossificans progressiva are distinctly different from those in patients with Klippel-Feil Syndrome. Clues from the BMP signaling pathway. Spine 30:1379–1385

47. Brarucha EP, Dastur HM (1964) Craniovertebral anomalies (a report of 40 cases). Brain 87:469–482

48. Wadia NH (1967) Myelopathy complicating congenital atlantoaxial dislocation (a study of 28 cases). Brain 90:449–472

49. Eck JC, Humphreys SC, Lim TH et al (2002) Biomechanical study on the effect of cervical spine on adjacent level intradiscal pressure and segmental motion. Spine 27:2431–2434

50. Tracy MR, Dormans JP, Kusumi K (2004) Klippel-Feil syndrome: clinical features and current understanding of etiology. Clin Orthop Rel Res 424: 183–190

51. Frobin W, Leivseth G, Biggemann M et al (2002) Sagittal plane segmental motion of the cervical spine. A new precision measurement protocol. Clin Biomech 17:21–31

52. Villas C (1984) Sinostosis cervicales y traumatismos en el esquí. In: Medicina De Montaña. Servicio de Publicaciones del Gobierno Vasco. Vitoria, pp 233–237

53. Garg A, Gaikwad SB, Gupta V et al (2004) Bipartite atlas with os odontoideum: case report. Spine 29: E224–E228

Tumors

15

Andreas F. Mavrogenis and Pietro Ruggieri

A small number of patients with neck pain may have a tumor in the cervical spine. Tumors of the axis (C2 vertebra) are rare [1, 2]. The location and unique structure of the upper cervical spine and proximity to vital structures make diagnosis and treatment difficult. Pain is usually the initial symptom; incidental diagnosis on plain radiographs is not uncommon [2, 3]. Spasm, kyphotic or scoliotic deformities, or torticollis, neck stiffness and dysphagia, neurological deficits, or spine instability may be associated symptoms [3–6].

15.1 Imaging

Plain radiographs may show a radiolucent and destructive lesion or severe osteopenia; pathological fracture, loss of a pedicle on an antero-posterior view, an osteoblastic lesion, bone destruction with preservation of the disks, paraspinal soft tissue mass with or without calcification, and collapse of the vertebral body with radiographic appearance of vertebra plana may be associated symptoms [1, 7, 8]. Computed tomography (CT) is more sensitive than plain films and more accurate than magnetic resonance imaging (MRI) for bone lesions; MRI is most useful for the diagnosis of intra- and extradural spinal lesions and soft tissue extension [5]. Bone scan shows increased uptake in the majority of spinal tumors. The disadvantage is the low specificity due to the high rates of false-positive findings in coexisting degenerative spondylosis in older patients. Additionally, in most cases, hemoproliferative tumors such as plasma cell dyscrasias produce little, if any, osteoblastic reaction and therefore are not evident on isotope bone scan [9].

15.2 Biopsy

CT-guided trocar biopsy can be performed successfully in the cervical spine, with low incidence of tumor spreading in the surrounding tissues [10]. Open incisional biopsy should be performed in cases where sufficient tissue is required; for anterior spine tumors, it is best obtained through an anterior approach rather than by laminectomy to avoid contamination of the epidural space [11]. Excisional biopsy should be reserved for tumors of the posterior elements of the cervical spine [12]. In few cases, when imaging features are strongly consistent with a certain diagnosis such as recurrent primary tumor, metastatic disease, and in cases in

A. F. Mavrogenis (✉)
First Department of Orthopaedics, Athens University Medical School, 41 Ventouri Street, 15562, Athens, Holargos, Greece
e-mail: afm@otenet.grandreasfmavrogenis@yahoo.gr

P. Ruggieri
Department of Orthopaedics, Istituto Ortopedico Rizzoli, University of Bologna, Bologna, Italy
e-mail: pietro.ruggieri@ior.it

D. S. Korres (ed.), *The Axis Vertebra*,
DOI: 10.1007/978-88-470-5232-1_15, © Springer-Verlag Italia 2013

Fig. 15.1 a Lateral radiograph and **b** axial computed tomography (CT) of the cervical spine of a 15-year-old male patient with osteoid osteoma of the axis

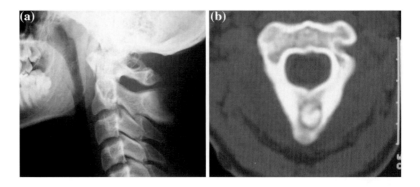

which a certain diagnosis such as multiple myeloma is obvious, biopsy can be avoided [12].

15.3 Benign Bone Tumors of the Axis

Approximately 10 % of osteoid osteomas occur in the spine. Upper cervical spine location is rare; however, osteoid osteoma is the most common benign bone tumor of the axis (Fig. 15.1) [2]. Most cases present before the age of 25 years [13–15]. Persistent cervical pain in an adolescent or young adult, frequently associated with radiation to the upper limb without specific dermatomal distribution, sometimes concomitant with muscle spasm is consistent with the diagnosis of osteoid osteoma [14, 15]. In contrast to extraspinal locations, only about one-third of patients respond to aspirin [14, 15]. Traditional treatment has been complete surgical removal of the nidus, with a recurrence rate of up to 4.5 % [16–18]. Percutaneous radiofrequency thermal ablation has been used successfully for the treatment for spinal osteoid osteomas without any complications from the spinal cord [19].

Aneurysmal bone cysts are the second most common benign bone tumors of the axis (Fig. 15.2) [2]. They more commonly affect females in the first two decades of life and involve the posterior neural arch [20–26]. Pain is the most frequent presenting symptom; spinal cord compression is possible as cyst grows [14]. Surgical treatment in the axis is difficult due to location and complex reconstruction [20, 21, 24,

27–30]; the local recurrence after curettage ranges from 5 to 10 % [20, 21, 23, 27, 28]. Embolization and percutaneous intralesional injection of calcitonin and methylprednisolone have been tried successfully for aneurysmal bone cysts of the upper cervical spine [25, 26]. However, both treatments require multiple sessions of therapy that take effect over the course of several months [25, 26]. In addition, embolization in the upper cervical spine is associated with the risk of spinal cord infarct [21] because the blood supply of the lesions is usually through branches of the vertebral artery [14, 24]. Radiation therapy may be necessary to reduce the risk of local recurrence [31, 32].

Osteoblastomas are the third most common benign tumors of the axis (Fig. 15.3) [2]. Although histologically identical to osteomas, osteoblastomas are much larger (>2 cm) and less common [14, 20]. Approximately 35 % occur in the spine [13–15]; about half of the cases occur in the lumbar spine, with the remaining equally distributed between the thoracic and cervical spine [14]. They most commonly arise from the posterior spinal elements, sometimes invading the vertebral body [14, 33–36]. Because of their slow growth and larger size, they tend to involve more than one element of the spine and usually manifest via local mass effect on adjacent structures and neurological deficits [14, 15, 37, 38]. Rarely, osteoblastomas may undergo sarcomatous changes [39]. Treatment for cervical spine osteoblastomas is complete surgical resection [14, 40]. Radiation therapy may be considered as adjuvant in patients with multiple recurrences [41].

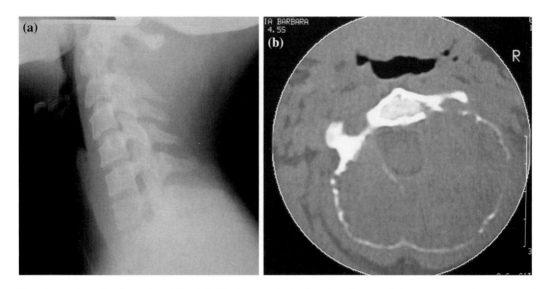

Fig. 15.2 **a** Lateral radiograph and **b** axial CT of the cervical spine of a 14-year-old female patient with aneurysmal bone cyst of the axis

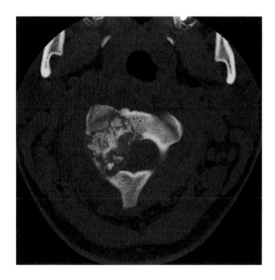

Fig. 15.3 Axial CT of the cervical spine of a 14-year-old female patient with osteoblastoma of the axis

Giant-cell tumor is the fourth most common benign tumor in the spine (1.4–9.4 %) (Fig. 15.4) [2, 42]; cervical location is as common as thoracic or lumbar [14, 43]. Spinal giant-cell tumor most commonly presents with pain due to the expansile lesion with or without vertebral collapse, spinal instability, and neurological deficits [43]. Preoperative embolization followed by marginal or intralesional resection and radiation therapy is usually the treatment of choice [7, 44–46]. Bone grafting should be avoided because the tumor is known to recur in the grafted bone [45, 46]. A 13.5 % risk of metastases of spinal giant-cell tumors compared with 1.8–9.1 % from other locations has been reported [47–50]. Local recurrence in the spine is reported to be lower compared with other locations [51].

Eosinophilic granuloma of the spine accounts for 6.5–25 % of all bone cases [14, 20, 52, 53]. The cervical spine is the third most common location after the thoracic and the lumbar spine [52–55]. Spinal location can be solitary or multiple and usually involves the vertebral body [14]. Cervical spine eosinophilic granuloma more often manifests with osteolytic lesions, rather than with vertebra plana [54]. In this setting, differential diagnosis with Ewing's sarcoma or lymphoma is necessary [14]. Eosinophilic granuloma may be self-limited and heal spontaneously [14]. Treatment for a painful, typical lesion with unique involvement of the vertebral body and absence of neurological deficits is conservative [54, 56, 57]. In patients with mild neurological deficits, immobilization and radiation have been used [58]. In patients with severe pain, restriction of motion, persistent

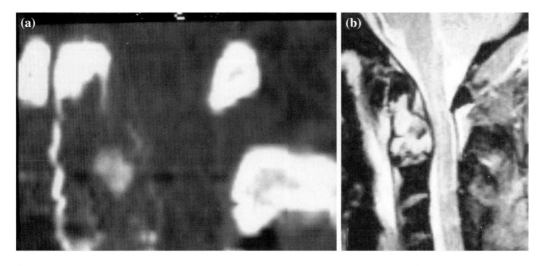

Fig. 15.4 Sagittal **a** CT and **b** T2-weighted magnetic resonance imaging (MRI) of the cervical spine of a 21-year-old male patient with giant-cell tumor of the axis

spinal subluxation, and/or neurological symptoms, surgical treatment is required [53–55, 59]. Chemotherapy should be reserved for systemic disease [54, 58, 59] and locations that preclude safe and complete excision [60]. Alternatively, computed tomography–guided intralesional methylprednisolone injection, as adjunct or primary treatment, has been safe and successful [61].

Fibromyxoma of bone is a rare benign fibrous tumor typically involving the jawbones [62]. Spinal location has been reported once (Fig. 15.5) [2]. Extragnathic lesions with abundant myxoid tissue have been designated as myxomas; in the presence of large amounts of differentiated fibrous tissue, they have been designated as fibromyxomas [1, 62–66]. Fibromyxoma should be distinguished from benign cartilage forming bone tumors such as chondromyxoid fibroma and myxoid chondrosarcoma from the absence of histological lobular pattern, chondroid matrix and variety of cells, and the more aggressive behavior of the latter. Association with myxoid fibrous dysplasia has also been implicated [1]. Pain is the typical presentation. The most common radiographic patterns are a well-defined radiolucent lesion with cortical destruction without periosteal reaction, an expansile central metaphyseal lesion with

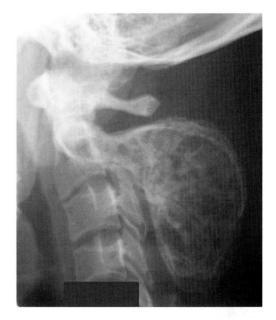

Fig. 15.5 Lateral radiograph of the cervical spine of a 21-year-old female patient with fibromyxoma of the axis

sclerotic rim, and a malignant lesion with ill-defined margins, cortical destruction, and soft tissue extension. An extraosseous mass has been reported in approximately one-third of cases. Complete curettage or excision is the treatment of choice [63, 65–67]; recurrence has been up to 13 % [63, 64].

15.4 Malignant Bone Tumors of the Axis

The occurrence and management of malignant bone tumors in the upper cervical spine are challenging [3, 4, 68]. In most cases, conservative, adjuvant, or palliative treatments including curettage and piecemeal tumor excision are only feasible because of the tumor extent and proximity to vital structures, resulting in high rates of local recurrences and distal metastases [68].

The spine is the most common site of bone metastases; in the axis, metastases are also the most common malignant lesions and the most common bone tumors overall (Fig. 15.6) [2]. Clinical symptoms develop due to increase in size of the lesion, compression of adjacent structures and nerve roots, spinal instability, and spinal cord compression [69]. Metastasis to the odontoid process is important because the mortality rate is >50 %, especially if

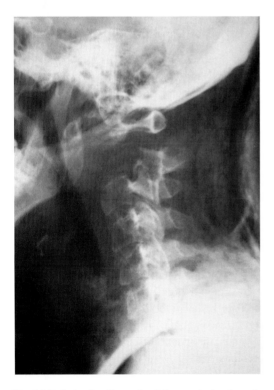

Fig. 15.6 Lateral radiograph of the cervical spine of a 44-year-old female patient with metastatic breast cancer of the axis

complicated with acute odontoid process fractures [70]. Depending on life expectancy, treatments of patients with cervical spine metastases include surgery, chemotherapy, and radiation therapy, depending on the stage of the disease and neurological impairment or instability. Percutaneous vertebroplasty can also be used for pain palliation [71]. However, bone metastases are progressive, even after combined surgical treatment and adjuvants, and the prognosis is poor [69–71].

Chordomas are low-grade, slow-growing, locally invasive malignant tumors from neoplastic transformation of notochordal remnants in the vertebral disks [68]. They account for 33 % of all primary malignant spinal tumors [72–74]; 50 % occur in the sacrum, 37 % in the clivus, and the others in decreasing order in the cervical (6 %), lumbar, and thoracic spine [1, 20, 68, 73, 74]. In the axis, chordomas are the third most common malignant bone tumors (Fig. 15.7) [2]. Chordomas metastasize late in their course [68]. They are more aggressive in children, showing high mitotic activity, hypercellularity and pleomorphism, and higher risk of metastatic spread [75, 76]. A long history of mild neck pain is the most common complaint, in addition to symptoms related to a slow-growing mass including dysphagia, upper respiratory obstruction, Horner's syndrome, and nerve root/cord compression [7]. En bloc surgical resection is the treatment of choice; however, excision is often limited by adjacent anatomic structures [68]. In most cases, only marginal or intralesional resection is feasible [77–80]. In these cases, recurrence has been 12–60 % [77, 80, 81] within 2–3 years, but can be as long as 10 years [82–84]. Chordomas are not sensitive to chemotherapy. Proton therapy and stereotactic radiation seem to slow the evolution of the disease and have 2- and 5-year local control rates of 82 and 50 %, respectively [3, 85–87].

Plasmacytoma and myeloma are the most common (30 %) primary malignant tumors of the spine; 3 % of the cases affect the cervical spine (Fig. 15.8) [1, 2]. Plasma cell neoplasms usually are radiosensitive even to low doses of conventional radiation. If neurological status is

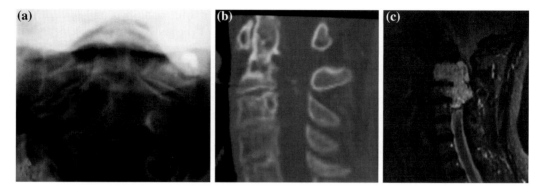

Fig. 15.7 **a** Anteroposterior radiograph (odontoid view), and sagittal **b** CT and **c** T2-weighted MRI of the cervical spine of a 67-year-old female patient with chordoma of the axis

Fig. 15.8 **a** Lateral tomography and **b** coronal CT of the cervical spine of a 28-year-old male patient with plasmacytoma of the axis

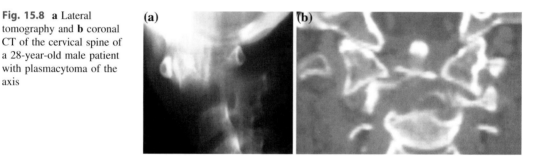

normal, the treatment of choice is radiation therapy with or without chemotherapy [3]. Surgical treatment is indicated in cases with progressive neurological deficits, spinal instability, nerve root/cord compression, or recurrences after maximum dose radiation [3, 9]. The prognosis for plasmacytoma is better than that for multiple myeloma [72]. Approximately 50 % of plasmacytomas will progress to multiple myeloma [2, 3, 85].

Osteosarcomas account for 10 % of primary malignant tumors of the spine [20, 36, 88, 89]; 0.5 % of cases affect the cervical spine [1]. In the upper cervical spine, osteosarcomas are the fourth most common malignant tumors; atlas involvement is more common than the axis [2]. Chemotherapy is the treatment of choice for osteosarcomas. Surgery should be regarded for palliation of advanced tumors. In cases of neurological deterioration, operative intervention for decompression and spinal stabilization may precede chemotherapy [89]. The natural course of

spinal osteosarcomas usually is rapid, with early lung metastases and a poor prognosis [3, 88].

Chondrosarcomas of the axis are rare (Fig. 15.9); 1.5 % of all chondrosarcomas affect the cervical spine [1–3]. Most are low-grade and relatively indolent and tend to recur locally before distant spreading occurs [90]. Chondrosarcomas are radiation and chemotherapy resistant [72]. The treatment of choice is wide-margin surgical resection. However, for chondrosarcomas of the upper cervical spine, piecemeal excision is frequently the only possible surgical procedure [3].

Epithelioid hemangioendothelioma of bone is a low-grade malignant endothelial tumor with a biologic behavior between that of hemangioma and angiosarcoma. Although it is the most common malignant vascular tumor of bone, it accounts for <1 % of all bone tumors [91]; spinal lesions account for <10 % of all cases [92]. Location in the axis is exceptional (Fig. 15.10) [2]. It may occur at any age; half of

Fig. 15.9 Sagittal CT of the cervical spine of a 67-year-old male patient with chondrosarcoma of the axis

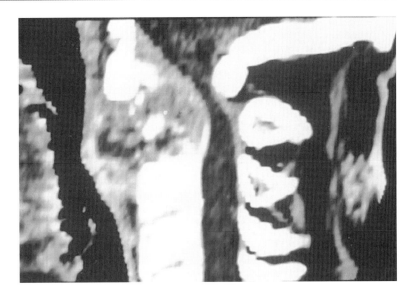

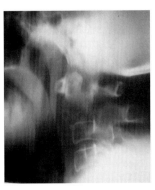

Fig. 15.10 Lateral tomography of the cervical spine of a 50-year-old male patient with hemangioendothelioma of the axis

the cases are seen in childhood or young adults. Characteristic feature is the tendency to multifocality [92, 93]. Localized pain and soft tissue swelling are the most common clinical symptoms [93, 94]. Treatment includes surgery, with or without adjuvant chemotherapy, radiation therapy, and embolization; recurrence has been up to 13 % [93, 94].

References

1. Unni KK (1996) Dahlin's bone tumors. General aspects and data on 11,087 cases, 5th edn. Lippincott-Raven, Philadelphia

2. Mavrogenis AF, Guerra G, Romantini M, Romagnoli C, Casadei R, Ruggieri P (2012) Tumours of the atlas and axis: a 37-year experience with diagnosis and management. Radiol Med 117(4):616–635
3. Boriani S, Sundaresan N, Weinstein JN (1998) Primary malignant tumors of the cervical spine. In: (ed) The cervical spine, 3rd edn. Lippincott-Raven, Philadelphia, pp 643–657
4. Abdu WA, Provencher M (1998) Primary bone and metastatic tumors of the cervical spine. Spine 23: 2767–2777
5. Papagelopoulos PJ, Mavrogenis AF, Currier BL et al (2004) Primary malignant tumors of the cervical spine. Orthopedics 27(10):1066–1077
6. Ilaslan H, Sundaram M, Unni KK (2003) Vertebral chondroblastoma. Skeletal Radiol 32(2):66–71
7. Boriani S, Weinstein JN, Biagini R (1997) Primary bone tumors of the spine. Terminology and surgical staging. Spine 22:1036–1044
8. Papagelopoulos PJ, Currier BL, Galanis E et al (2002) Vertebra plana caused by primary Ewing sarcoma: case report and review of the literature. J Spinal Disord Tech 15:252–257
9. McLain RF, Weinstein JN (1989) Solitary plasmacytomas of the spine: a review of 84 cases. J Spinal Disord 2:69–74
10. Brugieres P, Gaston A, Voisin MC et al (1992) CT-guided percutaneous biopsy of the cervical spine: a series of 12 cases. Neuroradiology 34:358–360
11. Hart RA, Boriani S, Biagini R et al (1997) A system for surgical staging and management of spine tumors. A clinical outcome study of giant cell tumors of the spine. Spine 22:1773–1783
12. Springfield DS, Rosenberg A (1996) Biopsy: complicated and risky. J Bone Joint Surg Am 78: 639–643
13. Rengachary SS, Sanan A (1998) Ivory osteoma of the cervical spine: case report. Neurosurgery 42:182–185

14. Levine AM, Boriani S (2005) Benign Tumors of the cervical spine. In: Clark CR, Benzel EC, Currier BL et al (eds) The cervical spine. Lippincott-Raven, Philadelphia, pp 816–839

15. Wang W, Kong L, Dong R et al (2006) Osteoma in the upper cervical spine with spinal cord compression. Eur Spine J 15(Suppl 5):616–620

16. Zileli M, Çagli S, Basdemir G, Ersahin Y (2003) Osteoid osteomas and osteoblastomas of the spine. Neurosurg Focus 15:1–6

17. Pettine KA, Klassen RA (1986) Osteoid osteoma and osteoblastoma of the spine. J Bone Joint Surg Am 68:354–361

18. Ozaki T, Liljenqvist U, Hillmann A et al (2002) Osteoid osteoma and osteoblastoma of the spine. Experiences with 22 patients. Clin Orthop Relat Res 397:394–402

19. Rybak LD, Gangi A, Buy X et al (2010) Thermal ablation of spinal osteoid osteomas close to neural elements: technical considerations. AJR Am J Roentgenol 195(4):W293–W298

20. Menezes AH (2008) Craniovertebral junction neoplasms in the pediatric population. Childs Nerv Syst 24(10):1173–1186

21. Boriani S, De Iure F, Campanacci L et al (2001) Aneurysmal bone cyst of the mobile spine: report on 41 cases. Spine (Phila Pa 1976) 26(1):27–35

22. Ozaki T, Halm H, Hillmann A, Shaffrey CI (1999) Aneurysmal bone cysts of the spine. Arch Orthop Trauma Surg 119:159–162

23. Papagelopoulos PJ, Currier BL, Shaughnessy WJ et al (1998) Aneurysmal bone cyst of the spine. Management and outcome. Spine 23:621–628

24. Bongioanni F, Assadurian E, Polivka M, George B (1996) Aneurysmal bone cyst of the atlas: operative removal through an anterolateral approach. A case report. J Bone Joint Surg Am 78:1574–1577

25. Gladden ML Jr, Gillingham BL, Hennrikus W, Vaughan LM (2000) Aneurysmal bone cyst of the first cervical vertebrae in a child treated with percutaneous intralesional injection of calcitonin and methylprednisolone. A case report. Spine 25:527–531

26. Mohit AA, Eskridge J, Ellenbogen R, Shaffrey CI (2004) Aneurysmal bone cyst of the atlas: successful treatment through selective arterial embolization: case report. Neurosurgery 55:982

27. Wang VY, Deviren V, Ames CP (2009) Reconstruction of C-1 lateral mass with titanium mesh cage after resection of an aneurysmal bone cyst of the atlas. J Neurosurg Spine 10(2):117–121

28. George B, Archilli M, Cornelius JF (2006) Bone tumors at the cranio-cervical junction. Surgical management and results from a series of 41 cases. Acta Neurochir (Wien) 148:741–749

29. George B, Dematons C, Cophignon J (1988) Lateral approach to the anterior portion of the foramen magnum. Application to surgical removal of 14 benign tumors: technical note. Surg Neurol 29:484–490

30. Menezes AH, Traynelis VC (2008) Anatomy and biomechanics of normal craniovertebral junction (a) and biomechanics of stabilization (b). Childs Nerv Syst 24(10):1091–1100

31. Combelles G, Delcambre B, Madelain M et al (1983) Le kyste anevrysmal rachidien. Considerations therapeutiques a propos de 6 observations. Neurochirurgie 29:1–11

32. Hay MC, Paterson D, Taylor TK (1978) Aneurysmal bone cysts of the spine. J Bone Joint Surg 60B(3):406–411

33. Nemoto O, Moser RP, Van Dam BE et al (1990) Osteoblastoma of the spine: review of 75 cases. Spine 15:1272–1280

34. Healey JH, Ghelman B (1986) Osteoid-osteoma and osteoblastoma: current concepts and recent advances. Clin Orthop Relat Res 204:76–85

35. Syklawer R, Osborn RE, Kerber CW et al (1990) MRI of vertebral osteoblastoma: report of two cases. Surg Neurol 34:421–426

36. Lopez-Barea F, Rodriguez-Peralto JL, Hernandez-Moneo JL et al (1994) Tumors of the atlas. 3 incidental cases of osteochondroma, benign osteoblastoma, and atypical Ewing's sarcoma. Clin Orthop Relat Res 307:182–188

37. Tarantino R, Piccirilli M, Anichini G, Delfini R (2008) Benign osteoblastoma of the odontoid process of the axis with secondary aneurysmal bone cyst component: a case report. Neurosurg Rev 31(1):111–115

38. Arvin B, Panchmatia JR, Casey AT (2009) Cervical C2 osteoma, unusual presentation and transoral approach for complete excision. Spine J 9(3):e9–e11

39. Amacher AL, Eltormey A (1985) Spinal osteoblastoma in children and adolescents. Childs Nerv Syst 1:29–32

40. Moore T, McLain RF (2005) Image-guided surgery in resection of benign cervicothoracic spinal tumors: report of two cases. Spine J 5:109–114

41. Shikata J, Yamamuro T, Hiokazu I et al (1987) Benign osteoblastoma of the cervical spine: a review of 75 cases. Surg Neurol 27:381–385

42. Sanjay BK, Sim FH, Unni KK et al (1993) Giant-cell tumours of the spine. J Bone Joint Surg Br 75-B:148–154

43. Biagini R, De Cristofaro R, Ruggieri P, Boriani S (1990) Giant-cell tumor of the spine: a case report. J Bone Joint Surg 72:1102–1107

44. Martin C, McCarthy EF (2010) Giant cell tumor of the sacrum and spine: series of 23 cases and a review of the literature. Iowa Orthop J 30:69–75

45. Di Lorenzo ND, Spallone A, Nolletti A, Nardi P (1980) Giant cell tumors of the spine: A clinical study of six cases, with emphasis on the radiological features, treatment and follow-up. Neurosurgery 6:29–34

46. Fidler MW (2001) Surgical treatment of giant cell tumours of the thoracic and lumbar spine: report of nine patients. Eur Spine J 10:69–77

47. Rock MG, Pritchard DJ, Unni KK (1984) Metastases from histologically benign giant cell tumor of bone. J Bone Joint Surg Am 66-A:269–274

48. Bertoni F, Present D, Sudanese A et al (1988) Giant-cell tumor of bone with pulmonary metastases. Six case reports and a review of the literature. Clin Orthop Relat Res 237:275–285

49. Kay RM, Eckardt JJ, Seeger LL et al (1994) Pulmonary metastasis of benign giant cell tumor of bone. Six histologically confirmed cases, including one of spontaneous regression. Clin Orthop Relat Res 302:219–230

50. McGough RL, Rutledge J, Lewis VO et al (2005) Impact severity of local recurrence in giant cell tumor of bone. Clin Orthop Relat Res 438:116–122

51. Sanerkin NG (1980) Malignancy, aggressiveness, and recurrence in giant cell tumor of bone. Cancer 46(7):1641–1649

52. Sweasey TA, Dauser RC (1989) Eosinophilic granuloma of the cervicothoracic junction. Case report. J Neurosurg 71:942–944

53. Tanaka N, Fujimoto Y, Okuda T et al (2005) Langerhans cell histiocytosis of the atlas. A report of three cases. J Bone Joint Surg Am 87(10): 2313–2317

54. Bertram C, Madert J, Eggers C (2002) Eosinophilic granuloma of the cervical spine. Spine 27:1408–1413

55. Dickinson LD, Farhat SM (1991) Eosinophilic granuloma of the cervical spine. A case report and review of the literature. Surg Neurol 35:57–63

56. Metellus P, Gana R, Fuentes S et al (2007) Spinal Langerhans' cell histiocytosis in a young adult: case report and therapeutic considerations. Br J Neurosurg 21(2):228–230

57. Yeom JS, Lee CK, Shin HY et al (1999) Langerhans' cell histiocytosis of the spine. Analysis of twenty-three cases. Spine 24:1740–1749

58. Osenbach RK, Youngblood LA, Menezes AH (1990) Atlanto-axial instability secondary to solitary eosinophilic granuloma of C2 in a 12-year-old girl. J Spinal Disord 3:408–412

59. Scarpinati M, Artico M, Artizzu S (1995) Spinal cord compression by eosinophilic granuloma of the cervical spine. Case report and review of the literature. Neurosurg Rev 18:209–212

60. Levy EI, Scarrow A, Hamilton RC et al (1999) Medical management of eosinophilic granuloma of the cervical spine. Pediatr Neurosurg 31(3):159–162

61. Rimondi E, Mavrogenis AF, Rossi G et al (2011) CT-guided corticosteroid injection for solitary eosinophilic granuloma of the spine. Skeletal Radiol 40(6):757–764

62. Dorfman HD, Czerniak B (1998) Bone Tumours. Mosby Inc., St. Louis

63. Marcove RC, Lindeque BG, Huvos AG (1989) Fibromyxoma of the bone. Surg Gynecol Obstet 169:115–118

64. Hardes J, Scheil-Bertram S, Gosheger G, Schulte M (2006) Fibromyxoma of bone: a case report and review of the literature. Acta Orthop Belg 72(1): 100–104

65. Adler CP (1981) Fibromyxoma of the femoral neck. J Cancer Res Clin Oncol 101:183–189

66. Sundaram M, Janney C, McDonald DJ (2000) Myxoma of the humerus: an exceptional site of origin. Skeletal Radiol 29:57–60

67. Abdelwahab FI, Hermann G, Klein MJ et al (1991) Fibromyxoma of bone. Skeletal Radiol 20:95–98

68. Fujita T, Kawahara N, Matsumoto T, Tomita K (1999) Chordoma in the cervical spine managed with en bloc excision. Spine 24:1848–1851

69. Harrington KD (1986) Metastatic disease of the spine. J Bone Joint Surg Am 68:1110–1115

70. Rayan F, Mukundan C, Shukla DD, Barrington RL (2009) Odontoid metastasis: a potential lethal complication. J Orthop Traumatol 10(4):199–201

71. Anselmetti GC, Manca A, Chiara G, Regge D (2009) Painful osteolytic metastasis involving the anterior and posterior arches of C1: percutaneous vertebroplasty with local anesthesia. J Vasc Interv Radiol 20(12):1645–1647

72. Sundaresan N, Krol G, Hughes JE (1990) Primary malignant tumors of the spine. In: Youmans JR (ed) Neurological Surgery, 3rd edn. WB Saunders Co, Philadelphia, pp 3548–3573

73. Huvos AG (1991) Bone tumors: diagnosis, treatment, and prognosis, 2nd edn. WB Saunders, Philadelphia, pp 599–624

74. Dahlin DC, MacCarthy CS (1952) Chordoma: a study of fifty-nine cases. Cancer 5:1170–1178

75. Borba LA, Mefty O AL, Mrak RE, Suen J (1996) Cranial chordomas in children and adolescents. J Neurosurg 84:584–591

76. Coffin CM, Swanson PE, Wick MR, Dehner LP (1993) Chordoma in childhood and adolescence. A clinicopathologic analysis of 12 cases. Arch Pathol Lab Med 117:927–933

77. Menezes AH, Gantz BJ, Traynelis VC, McCulloch TM (1997) Cranial base chordomas. Clin Neurosurg 44:491–509

78. Boriani S, Chevalley F, Weinstein JN et al (1996) Chordoma of the spine above the sacrum. Treatment and outcome in 21 cases. Spine 21:1569–1577

79. Forsyth PA, Cascino TL, Shaw EG et al (1993) Intracranial chordomas: a clinicopathological and prognostic study of 51 cases. J Neurosurg 78: 741–747

80. Gay E, Sekhar LN, Rubinstein E et al (1995) Chordomas and chondrosarcomas of the cranial base: results and follow-up of 60 patients. Neurosurgery 36:887–896

81. Watkins L, Khudados ES, Kaleoglu M et al (1993) Skull base chordomas: a review of 38 patients, 1958–88. Br J Neurosurg 7:241–248

82. Austin JP, Urie MM, Cardenosa G, Munzenrider JE (1993) Probable causes of recurrence in patients with chordoma and chondrosarcoma of the base of skull and cervical spine. Int J Radiat Oncol Biol Phys 25:439–444

83. Benk V, Liebsch NJ, Munzenrider JE et al (1995) Base of skull and cervical spine chordomas in children treated by high-dose irradiation. Int J Radiat Oncol Biol Phys 31:577–581

84. Fagundes MA, Hug EB, Liebsch NJ et al (1995) Radiation therapy for chordomas of the base of skull and cervical spine: patterns of failure and outcome after relapse. Int J Radiat Oncol Biol Phys 33:579–584

85. Marucci L, Niemierko A, Liebsch NJ et al (2004) Spinal cord tolerance to high-dose fractionated 3D conformal proton-photon irradiation as evaluated by equivalent uniform dose and dose volume histogram analysis. Int J Radiat Oncol Biol Phys 59:551–555

86. Noël G, Feuvret L, Calugaru V et al (2005) Chordomas of the base of the skull and upper cervical spine. One hundred patients irradiated by a 3D conformal technique combining photon and proton beams. Acta Oncol 44(7):700–708

87. Debus J, Schulz-Ertner D, Schad L et al (2000) Stereotactic fractionated radiotherapy for chordomas and chondrosarcomas of the skull base. Int J Radiat Oncol Biol Phys 47:591–596

88. Shives TC, Dahlin DC, Sim FH et al (1986) Osteosarcoma of the spine. J Bone Joint Surg Am 68:660–668

89. Hart RA, Weinstein JN (1995) Primary benign and malignant musculoskeletal tumors of the spine. Semin Spine Surg 7:288–302

90. Shives TC, McLeod RA, Unni KK, Schray MF (1989) Chondrosarcoma of the spine. J Bone Joint Surg Am 71:1158–1165

91. Roessner A, Boehling T (2002) Angiosarcoma. In: Fletcher CDM, Unni KK, Mertens F (eds) World Health Organization classification of tumours of soft tissue and bone. Pathology and genetics of tumours of soft tissue and bone. IARC Press, Lyon, pp 322–323

92. Aflatoon K, Staals E, Bertoni F et al (2004) Hemangioendothelioma of the spine. Clin Orthop Relat Res 418:191–197

93. Campanacci M, Boriani S, Giunti A (1980) Hemangioendothelioma of bone: a study of 29 cases. Cancer 46:804–814

94. Marks DS, Thomas AM, Thompson AG et al (1995) Surgical management of haemangioendothelioma of the spine. Eur Spine J 4:186–190

Index

D. S. Korres (ed.), *The Axis Vertebra*,
DOI: 10.1007/978-88-470-5232-1, © Springer-Verlag Italia 2013